Coping with Chronic Pain

Coping with Chronic Pain

by Nelson H. Hendler, M.D.

and Judith Alsofrom Fenton

Clarkson N. Potter, Inc./Publishers

DISTRIBUTED BY CROWN PUBLISHERS, INC., NEW YORK

Inquiries should be addressed to

Clarkson N. Potter, Inc.
One Park Avenue,
New York, N.Y. 10016

Printed in the United States of America
Published simultaneously in Canada by
General Publishing Company Limited

Designed by A Good Thing, Inc.

Library of Congress Cataloging in Publication Data

Hendler, Nelson.
Coping with chronic pain.

Bibliography: p.
1. Pain—Psychological aspects. 2. Pain—Prevention.
I. Fenton, Judith Alsofrom, joint author.
II. Title. [DNLM: 1. Chronic disease—Popular works.
2. Pain—Popular works. WL704 H497c]
BF515.H46 1979   616'.047   78-21284
ISBN 0-517-53440-1

To Lee, Sam and Alex
who are all joy to me—
N.H.

To Rick, my inspiration—
J.A.F.

Contents

Foreword

In my own life I have experienced pain, and I am aware of how it altered my life-style, as well as the stress that I experienced as a result of it. Most recently, I suffered pain in both hips that progressed from the mere annoyance of discomfort to a fully developed pain-encumbered existence. It is common knowledge that certain individuals may be "driven to drink" or become subject to various toxicomanias (narcotic or tranquilizer abuse or addiction) as a result of stressful life situations or constant pain, but I successfully avoided these pitfalls by adhering to basic philosophical tenets advanced in my book *Stress Without Distress.*[1] Recognizing I could not overcome or correct the pain, I utilized the concepts of altruistic egoism, adaptability, and syntoxic behavior (being at one with the environment). I was able to rely on people to help me physically by not being too proud to ask for help, but functioning, personally, with a code of mutual assistance that enabled me to freely offer help and receive help without rancor. I was not resentful of the physical aid provided by others when I was crippled by my hips, because I was adaptable—I recognized my limitations and accepted them. I did not avoid stress, despite the pain; but I conserved my energies for more productive work rather than fighting or resenting the pain—thus I became syntoxic in my behavior. This helped me cope with the pain and disability until I could have my offending hips replaced with artificial ones, as shown in my book *The Stress of My Life.*[2] I now can get around far better than before the operation, with much less pain, but as a reminder of my experiences I keep one of the offending hip bones (head of the femur) in a jar of formaldehyde on a shelf in my office. I delight in scolding the bone each day, reminding it of all the pain and stress it caused me, and how it must remain embalmed forever as its punishment.

However, not all people can understand and cope with pain the way I could, probably because they have little knowledge about it. It is a difficult sensation to comprehend, although much has been written about it by physiologists, neurologists, psychologists, psychiatrists, neurosurgeons, anesthesiologists, and others. Pain is a stressor—the most complex and least understood stressor—despite illusions to the contrary. Cannon's classic papers on the effects of pain, hunger, fear, and rage on sympathetic activity and epinephrine (EP) secretion stimulated many subsequent studies. Somatic pain and mental pain (grief) have been regarded as paradigms of stressors of considerable importance, particularly in man and higher animals. Attempts to measure pain, employing dolorimeters, using noxious stimulilike heat, electrical stimulation, and even lasers, are imperfect, because the same degree of stimulation may cause different intensities of pain, depending upon a variety of conditioning factors that determine somatic-pain sensitivity. Pavlov was well aware of these distinctions and sought to demonstrate how training (conditioning) could alter an animal's response to a particular stimulus. Furthermore, the great degree of variations in response among various animals does not help in the quantitative assessment of the indicators that can be considered as truly nonspecific and, hence, as stress effects. (A great many stimuli will produce the same physiological response, with secretion of the same hormones, and therefore can be considered nonspecific responses.) Still, it has been clearly established that physical pain can increase the secretion of the "stress" hormone cortisol, reduce white blood cells that fight infection, and change the brain-wave pattern of EEG recordings. Some of the investigators feel that they can differentiate the body's response to pain from other types of stressor effects, but they did not consider the concept of the nonspecific nature of the stress response of the body. However, its manifestations cannot be the same in all cases, because of the diverse conditioning agents that always influence it.[3]

I first met Dr. Hendler in Chicago in May 1978 at the request of my friend Dr. Joel Elkes, who serves on my Board of Directors of the International Institute of Stress, in Montreal. At that time we talked of forming the American Institute of Stress and further discussed Dr. Hendler's experiences with research in the field of pain and stress. I was delighted to learn that he was a third-generation student of two outstanding physiologists, having himself been trained by Dr. William Blake, a student of Cannon's, and by Dr. Horsley Gantt, a student of Pavlov's. Additionally, he had been a resident in psychiatry when Dr. Elkes was chairman of the Department of Psychiatry in Behavioral Medicine at the Johns Hopkins University School of Medicine. As we talked, it was apparent to me, in light of my own experiences, that his grasp of the effect of pain and suffering is most accurate. He also has a fine background in neurophysiology and neuroendocrinology, which is most useful in the understanding of the basic mechanisms of pain and ways of coping with it—ranging from the appropriate use of pharmacological agents to group therapy. Indeed, this broadbased, multifactorial approach is the only way to treat pain, since it is virtually impossible to dissect the various physiological, psychological, and pharmacological components of this most complex sensation. I was delighted to have the opportunity to read this book, and I am certain that other readers who have experienced pain and suffering will greatly appreciate the comprehensive nature of the material, as well as the technical excellence of this work. Indeed, Dr. Hendler is what I call the "Famulus" (the ideal pupil and assistant) to a variety of "Faustian" teachers (ideal teachers and chiefs). [4] A while ago I gave Dr. Hendler my book *From Dream to Discovery,* and I trust that he will fulfill the progression of evolving from a Famulus type to a Faustian type as he progresses through the necessary steps of research.[4] I wish him every luck and success in his pursuits.

Hans Selye, C.C., M.D., Ph.D., D.Sc.
President—The Hans Selye International Institute of Stress

1. Selye, Hans. *Stress Without Distress.* Philadelphia and New York: J. B. Lippincott Company, 1974, pp. 128–31.
2. ———. *The Stress of My Life.* Toronto: McClelland & Stewart, Ltd., 1977, pp. 128–60 (photographs).
3. ———. *Stress in Health and Disease.* Boston and London: Butterworths, 1976, pp. 200–201.
4. ———. *From Dream to Discovery.* New York, Toronto, London: McGraw-Hill Book Company, 1964, pp. 28–29.

Preface

My interest in the problem of chronic pain began a number of years ago, when, as a third-year resident in psychiatry at the Johns Hopkins Hospital, I was assigned to the psychiatric liaison service. The service provided psychiatric consultations to patients in a general hospital, and I soon learned that of all the patients I had to deal with at that time, the ones I felt most poorly equipped to handle were those who complained of chronic pain. I turned to a supervisor and good friend, Dr. Tom Wise, for advice. Dr. Wise, who is currently chairman of the Department of Psychiatry at Fairfax County Hospital in Falls Church, Virginia, recommended that I read a number of articles on the psychology and pharmacology of chronic pain. However, after reviewing these papers, it was apparent to me that I was not the only physician to have been confounded by the treatment of chronic-pain patients. Most of the articles offered such farfetched psychological interpretations that, in my wildest imagination, I could not conceive of how they could have any validity when applied to the people I had seen. The papers addressing the pharmacology and treatment of chronic pain were as unilluminating as those dealing exclusively with the psychology of pain.

The problem, I was to learn, is that physicians, who are all carefully trained in the treatment of acute pain, make the mistake of applying these same principles to their understanding and treatment of chronic-pain patients. This approach invites disaster—to apply the remedies of acute pain to someone whose pain is of longer, perhaps indefinite, duration, can often lead to addiction to a variety of drugs, such as Valium, Demerol, Talwin, Dalmane, Phenobarbitol, and Percodan, to name just a few. These drugs are freely dispensed by well-intentioned doctors, whose only concern is helping the patient. Yet, the very end they seek is offset by the problems engendered by the inappropriate use of drugs.

The anguish of chronic pain is a two-way street. The patient who has not responded to surgery or medications, and who is misunderstood by those who treat him, causes many problems for his family and physicians. His disorder is not visible or measurable by standard indicators, and still his complaints persist, placing his doctors and relations at a loss for the proper response. Because chronic pain does not show up on X-rays or electrical tests and is not manifested by a fever or a broken limb, it is often ascribed to psychological origins. The victim of chronic pain must learn to live with the disdain and disbelief, or at the very least, lack of sympathy, of those who are closest to him. It was this kind of prejudice that led me to a more thorough investigation of the problem.

It was fortunate that my interest in chronic pain developed while I was at Johns Hopkins Hospital, where there is a Chronic Pain Treatment Center under the excellent guidance of Dr. Donlin Long, chairman of the Department of Neurosurgery. Dr. Long has both a doctorate in anatomy and an M.D., and his understanding of chronic pain and the anatomical aspect of this disorder is extraordinary—and far different from most physicians'. In addition, Dr. Long's vast clinical experience as a surgeon and a neurosurgeon dealing specifically with chronic pain makes him uniquely qualified to treat this problem. Because of my research background in neurophysiology, both Dr. Long and Dr. Wise suggested that I serve as the psychiatric consultant at the Chronic Pain Treatment Center. All three of us recognized that this would be a trial by fire, since so little was known about the chronic-pain patient from a psychiatric and pharmacological point of view. I saw it as a challenge and an opportunity to add to our knowledge and understanding of chronic pain—an opportunity I did not want to miss.

For the first two years I floundered around, noting the distress of some patients, hearing of pain's awesome toll on their families, friends, and personal lives. I also observed patients who did not experience this same degree of distress. After several years it was apparent to me that there were three broad categories of chronic pain patients: those who had psychiatric problems as a result of their chronic pain; those who, from whatever motivation, utilized their chronic pain to their advantage and those people who responded to the stress of chronic pain by fighting back and working around the discomfort. (There may be a fourth group: those who have chronic pain but have never come to the attention of the physician.) I also observed the prejudice expressed toward these patients—by nurses, physicians, employers, and family. It seemed to me that what was needed was a clear-cut structure and set of guidelines for physicians, family, and friends of chronic-pain patients. Also, it was apparent that the patients themselves could benefit from a fuller understanding of the process they were experiencing. This is the void that I felt needed to be filled and that led to some of the research and observations on which this book is based.

At that time there was no satisfactory diagnostic system for both medical and psychiatric explanations of chronic pain, and so I began to develop a simple system for categorizing chronic-pain patients. I constructed a preliminary framework, based on 315 patients, for understanding the problems these pain victims experience; this also gave rise to some ideas for the treatment of their affliction. Now, after an additional three years at the Chronic Pain Treatment Center, during which time I have seen nearly 2,000 patients, I have found several flaws within the new diagnostic outline, but by and large it has proved a useful tool for most physicians associated with the treatment of chronic pain. A screening test I developed is now used in a more refined form at Johns Hopkins Hospital to help categorize chronic-pain patients and to decide on the type of treatment that can be most effectively applied to each case. The screening test has also shown itself to be a useful means of predicting responses to surgical procedures for the relief of chronic pain, of preventing unnecessary surgery, and of helping to select those patients who can benefit from surgery and who otherwise might not have been chosen. It is most gratifying to me that we are now able to provide a degree of specificity in the diagnosis of patients with chronic pain.

I hope that this book will serve to educate physicians, family members, and patients themselves about chronic pain. I have learned quite a bit from my patients, and this my coauthor, Judy Alsofrom Fenton, and I have tried to pass on to our readers. One lesson I have been taught—and exposed to repeatedly—is that chronic pain is a disease affecting all members of the family unit. I tell my patients that "you don't have a pain—your entire family has a pain." Victims of chronic pain complain of marital difficulties, trouble with their children, and strained social relations with relatives and friends. Our goal in *Coping with Chronic Pain* is to make this problem less mysterious and less frightening and to point out some steps that the pain victim, his doctors, and family can take to find help—or that the pain victim can take to help himself.

Nelson H. Hendler, M.D.
Stevenson, Maryland

Acknowledgments

This author is grateful to many people who have assisted with the compilation of this book. Of especial note are Drs. Donlin Long and Tom Wise. Dr. Wise provided much of the reference material, clinical guidance, and moral support I needed during the early phases of my experience with chronic-pain patients, while Dr. Long continues to dazzle me with his knowledge and interpretation of symptoms, his grasp of neuroanatomy, and his insight into patients. Dr. Long and I have worked together on many chronic-pain patients, and I have developed a deep admiration and respect for the man. I have learned more clinical medicine on rounds with him than I ever could imagine, and I am delighted with my five-year association with the Chronic Pain Treatment Center at Johns Hopkins Hospital. I also would like to thank Judy Alsofrom Fenton, who has the amazing ability to absorb massive amounts of incomprehensible medical data, digest them, and assemble them into a most readable form. Also, it has been a pleasure to work with Nancy Novogrod of Clarkson N. Potter Inc./Publishers, for she has made the completion of this book a nearly painless delivery. Above all, I want to thank my wife, Lee, and our two sons, Sam and Alex, for their understanding and support.

However, the real authors of this book are the many chronic-pain patients I have known over the past five years, since they have taught me more about chronic pain than all the physicians and textbooks combined. They are the *raison d'être* for this work.

Authors' Note

Because the English language has yet to come up with a pronoun that expresses both the male and female gender as one word in the third person, we have used the conventional "he" when referring to a person of an undesignated sex.

All the case histories contained in this book are based on factual diagnoses, but the characters and their lives are purely fictional. Any similarity to persons living or dead is purely coincidental.

Coping with Chronic Pain

Introduction

Pain: the kind you wake up with; the kind that stays with you until you fall asleep. This is chronic pain. It can nag a person off and on for as little as six months or for as long as a dozen or more years. Some physicians speculate that there are more than enough victims to make chronic pain the nation's third largest health problem, after cancer and heart disease. It is certainly the country's most underrated health problem—bar none.

This book is about what chronic pain is and how to cope with it. You will learn that, unlike any other pain, chronic pain has no apparent meaning and no real hope of an end in sight, whereas the pain of a cut or ruptured appendix is a useful warning that something is amiss. This kind of pain stops when corrective measures have been taken, and it usually never returns again.

This book, though, will not tell you about any magic cures. There are none. In fact, you will learn that securing relief can be hard work, and treatment will be both emotionally and physically demanding. You will discover that you are not alone, that there are doctors and other people willing to assist you in the search for what seems to be an elusive goal—freedom from pain. Also, you will learn to cope with chronic pain: included are exercises and special behavioral techniques that you can practice on your own and that will help change your attitude so you can live without pain being the focus of your life.

Coping with chronic pain also means learning all about it, understanding the enemy in order to squelch it. Where does chronic pain come from? How does it start? Can it be stopped? This book will tell you, in terms that you can understand, about pain and its place in the body's nervous systems, how the nervous systems work, how these systems send pain messages to the brain. Pain messages also can be interrupted, halted in their tracks. You will learn that you *can* stop the pain, and so can your doctor, and that relief is in sight.

Throughout the book, chronic pain will be referred to as a disease, not a symptom of something else. This is one of the keys to successfully treating chronic-pain sufferers. You will find out about all the latest approaches to the treatment of chronic pain; these include exercises you can do at home, advice on how to work more effectively with your doctor, and the specialized pain clinics that are located in several places across the country in medical centers, hospitals, and annexes to physicians' offices.

If you suffer from any form of chronic pain, you will learn that you have a lot of company. If you have low back pain, for example, your fellow sufferers number in the millions. Hundreds of thousands of people suffer from arthritis, bursitis, tennis elbow, and housemaid's knee. There are thousands afflicted with causalgia, a searing pain often resulting from a shock to the nervous system; there are neuralgia victims; and there are victims of phantom limb pain, which sometimes attacks an amputee years after the limb is gone. In this book we will discuss all these problems, along with toothaches, earaches, excruciating migraine headaches, the difficult pain of terminal cancer caused by the blockage of organs by tumor growth or the out and out destruction of the tissues by the disease.

You will learn about depression and anxiety, chronic pain's partners in making you feel bad. These and other related emotions, such as frustration, anger, self-pity, and fear, can cause their own type of pain and contribute to a vicious pain circle. Say your nagging stabbing pain begins in the morning, and you take some medication for it that offers a temporary respite. By afternoon you may begin to tense up from anxiety brought on by the anticipation of pain, the fear that it will return before you are supposed to take your pills again. The anxiety produces tension, which causes your muscles to ache and your head to throb. You begin to feel depressed—your life seems to be ruled by pain and pills.

Pain affects how you treat people and how they treat you. It defines your life-style. It has become your master. When the pain appears to have affected the way other people treat you, you find yourself being attacked by it all the more. You are dogged by it; pain, anxiety, and more pain have got you in a stranglehold. This book will explain how you can escape. You will see how chronic pain can mold your personality; how homelife, ethnic background, social status, and even your paycheck all can be components of your pain; and you will learn how to build a defense.

Scientists have invented new techniques and devices to help pain sufferers cope as well as adapting old techniques or old equipment and using them in new ways to relieve pain. You will learn what devices to block pain messages—acupuncture, surgery, biofeedback, hypnosis, and group therapy—require of you, their pros and cons, what they can do for you, and which one(s) are suitable to your pain.

Drugs, too, are part of the weaponry in the war against pain. Though most physicians or pain-clinic staff would prefer to see their patients drug free, certain types of pain can best be managed with drugs. How these drugs work will also be discussed.

You may find your problem described in this book or you may recognize the pain that a friend or relative has described to you. Some answers may be of help to you now, or sometime in the future.

Most important, after reading this book we hope you will be well informed enough to know that when someone says "it hurts," the problem may not be as simple as it sounds.

Myths About Chronic Pain

- It's all in your head.
- If you ignore it, the pain will go away.
- Nobody ever felt as bad as you.
- You did something wrong in the past; you deserve the pain you have now.
- Pain is the result of abusing your body.
- All pain is the same.
- You look so good! How can you have chronic pain?
- You can learn to live with it.
- You feel better if you see someone worse off than you.
- Medical science can cure anything.
- I won't have to live with this the rest of my life.
- My pain is my own.
- The doctors don't care.
- Pain medicine will help my chronic pain.

1
Do You Have Chronic Pain?
What Is It and How Is It Different from Other Pain

Pain is a subjective experience; it is a personal possession, a private feeling, and as individual as a fingerprint. It can be acute or chronic. *Acute pain* is a message to its victim. The brain receives so many messages in a single day that you may miss completely some of the transmissions.

Pulling tangles out of your hair in the morning may cause you some very short-term acute pain. Burning your finger on a hot mug of coffee during breakfast may produce some longer lasting pain. You may twist your ankle while running to catch a commuter train and feel uncomfortable from both the soreness in your ankle and from being out of breath. A hangnail may annoy you all day, or your corns may start acting up because you wore tight shoes. And if your boss yells at you or your children demand a lot from you, a headache may be your reward at day's end. All of these aches and stings and burns are pain messages.

Yet all of these pains are relatively easy to handle. They are short-lived, and you don't have to worry about them—you can pinpoint their source if you notice them at all. The yanked hair, the twisted ankles, the aching corns are all examples of *acute* pain.

Acute pain is generally sharp and short. It carries a warning that has a time limit. It tells you that something is wrong in some part of your body and immediate corrective action is necessary. The time limit can be the instant that it takes to pull a comb through a knot in your hair or the time needed for a broken bone to mend. Acute pain lasts at most for about two months.

Acute pain, therefore, has a protective function. Whether it is the result of trauma—a bodily injury produced by violence or an outside agent such as fire or chemicals—or the result of a disorder of the body's pain-producing mechanisms—such disorders would be lesions on nerves that send or receive pain messages—acute pain acts as a signal for the body to take action.

Because it is a subjective experience, pain is not purely a physical phenomenon that occurs somewhere in the mysterious recesses of the body. There are psychological components as well. These components, no less important than the physical, usually come into play when the pain no longer functions as a protective mechanism, when it has passed from acute to chronic. Time provides the basic distinction between acute and chronic. While the experience of pain is always subjective and personal, when it lasts through six months or more of periodic or unremitting episodes, pain can be decisively defined as *chronic.*

Whereas acute pain can be readily tied to a source, the sources of chronic pain are often uncertain. Whereas acute pain can be called a symptom of a wound, a burn, a fracture, a collapsed lung, chronic pain is more correctly described as a disease itself, rather than a symptom of something else. But it is a complex disease, which often has an underlying organic cause that is nearly impossible to detect.

For this reason one of the biggest problems for chronic-pain patients is getting someone to believe that they actually are in pain. Few people who have not experienced pain that persists for more than six months, let alone years, can believe that anyone could live with it that long. The chronic pain coupled with this lack of understanding causes many patients to find life unbearable and entertain thoughts of suicide.

How, then, do these millions of chronic-pain sufferers get someone to believe them, to give them relief? Listen to this woman who went to a clinic that treats pain patients. She is in a therapy session with fellow sufferers.

She sits quietly to the side of the circle of people. Tears are slowly falling down her cheeks. The group leader notices her and asks her what's wrong. She can't seem to answer him, but her face and neck turn red and she sheds a few more tears. The leader once more quietly asks her to explain her behavior or tell the group what she is feeling. She says she hurts. She tells the room full of strangers that the pain is slowly killing her, that it is destroying her life, ruining her relationship with her husband. No one cares about her anymore and no one in her family or neighborhood wants to talk with her anymore, because all she can talk about, it seems, is her pain. The pain is horrible, she tells the group. It's like a knife twisting deeper and deeper inside her neck, never ending. Some heads nod in sympathy and agreement, and her tears stop flowing, for a while.

The woman is telling her therapy group about her chronic pain—a pain in her neck that has hounded her for nearly four years. Each member of her group seems to understand, at least a little, for they are all afflicted with their own chronic pain.

Pain is a universally distressing feeling, whether acute or chronic. Both man and animal are liable to feel pain during the course of their lives. Yet while animals are limited to screeching or crying in pain, the vocabulary of pain for humans is more complex. The words that describe pain differ from person to person.

It hurts, it feels bad. It's uncomfortable. It feels like there's a knife slowly twisting in my back. It's a stabbing pain. It feels numb. It's a prickly sensation. It feels awful. It burns. It feels like pins and needles. It's like an elephant sitting on my chest. It feels sore. It's a searing pain. It stings. It's simply unbearable. These phrases could all be describing a pulled back muscle, a sinus headache, or an aching limb.

But these are just a few of the phrases used to express pain. They can be describing a sentiment, a physical sensation, or an emotion. It's easy to see why so many physicians fail to diagnose chronic pain or to trace it back to its source—they simply don't know what their patients are talking about. It's also easy to see that the communication of pain can cause a psychological problem for the chronic-pain sufferer. The person with acute pain can point to his broken leg and say what's bothering him, but the person with chronic pain, pain whose origins are less defined, pain that lingers on in time—that person is not understood by his family, his friends, or even his own doctor. What is so obvious to the chronic-pain sufferer, a dull ache that continually destroys his sleep, is invisible to others and, what's almost worse, may not seem to be a serious problem to other people.

Another problem for chronic-pain sufferers is that their pain generally cannot be measured or tested for with readily available diagnostic equipment. A hidden pain, for which no clear remedy can be prescribed, can evolve into a life-style for some people. Just like the junkie whose habit dictates a life-style of hustling for money, shooting up drugs, and then nodding out from their effect, for some sufferers chronic pain can come to dictate when they get up in the morning, what they do during the day, and when they fall asleep at night. Many chronic-pain victims have unconsciously hopped on a merry-go-round existence with the hope of grabbing not a brass ring but anything that will stop the constant pain.

If you suffer from chronic pain, you may have hopped on the chronic pain merry-go-round at your bathroom chest. You were looking for the aspirin bottle. After all, doesn't every doctor seem to say at one time or another "Take two aspirin and call me in the morning" for almost any illness? In your case, the pain did not go away in the morning.

So you took your pain to your local pharmacist and asked him to recommend something. He suggested a commercial remedy slightly stronger than aspirin. Since you told him that the pain kept waking you at night (or sometimes prevented you from getting to sleep at all), the druggist also suggested a mild, over-the-counter sedative. You tried these nonprescription drugs for a while, but they did not work at all.

Without sleep, you became irritable. With nothing readily available at the marketplace that might stop your pain, you decided it was time to see a doctor. You tried to tell him what was wrong. He couldn't see or feel anything out of the ordinary, he said. He took tests, ordered X-rays, poked and prodded, and asked you how it felt when he tapped you here and there. He asked you where it hurt. You told him, he listened.

Finally, the doctor wrote a prescription for a pain killer, a mild analgesic. You tried it for a time, took it faithfully on schedule. It seemed to make some of the pain ease up, but it made you groggy. You went back to your doctor with these complaints, and in his desire to help you get over the pain, he prescribed a slightly stronger analgesic, perhaps with a narcotic base. He also may have prescribed something to make you more alert during the day. But you were so alert, you could not get to sleep at night, so you started gulping down sleeping pills left over from another illness. You ate them like candy. Soon, you were carrying around what seemed like a shopping bag filled with rainbow-colored pills and capsules—but you still were carrying your pain, too.

If you had the time, money, and stamina you went to several

doctors, looking for one who possessed the magic pill, one who would give you the relief you were after that very first time you reached for the aspirin bottle in your medicine chest. All the doctors prescribed more pills—to no avail. Eventually you had sought out the best advice in your community; there was nobody left to give you any new ideas. They said they had done all they could for you.

You were desperate, willing to try anything, spend everything. Through the friend of a friend, you were referred to a surgeon who, when you made the appointment, said he might be able to help you, no guarantees. He had helped other people with similar conditions, similar complaints. Maybe he said he would cut something; maybe he told you he would take something out. You were willing to risk an operation, several operations, anything to get rid of the pain.

The pain might have disappeared after the surgeon's scalpel made its mark, but if it didn't no one believed that you still could be in any kind of pain, especially after all those years and all that money spent looking for a cure.

Unfortunately, in some cases relief from this life-style, relief from chronic pain, may paradoxically bring on another illness: depression. Some scientists suggest that it can replace physical suffering as a focus for all thought and a determinant for all activity. This phenomenon is called replacement depression, and it attacks people who actually need their chronic pain, to whom the pain has become a useful part of everyday life. The person who has to convince himself that there is a reason he is unable to work, to perform to standards, to have good sex with a spouse; the whiplash victim who heals sooner than his insurance claim is settled, or anyone who has come to use his chronic pain as proof that he's alive—something like pinching yourself to prove that you are not dreaming—is a likely candidate for this syndrome. Take the chronic pain away and you are taking away his security blanket. You may cause him to become depressed.

This replacement depression is similar to a depression seen in victims of brainwashing or survivors of concentration camps. These victims and survivors had adjusted to a way of life: they depended on the routine of abuse and harassment as a stabilizing element in their otherwise chaotic life. They adjusted their feelings, activities, even instincts for survival to that way of life. A sudden change in the routine, even if it led to an improvement, imposed unexpected distress and stress. This stress, in turn, led to depression, or even psychiatric breakdowns. The same holds true for the chronic-pain patient suddenly "deprived" of his pain. His routine is changed, there is stress in adjusting to a new way of life, and depression sets in.

Chronic pain itself may be addictive. Some scientific studies have shown that brain pathways that carry a great many pain messages come to expect them and carry the chronic-pain messages even if they are no longer sent by the original source (like a computer that continues to send a bill long after it is paid).

Chronic pain can attack anyone. How long it lasts and how it feels—dull, sharp, stinging—differs from person to person. Chronic pain is a personal perception, an individual experience, and it is real. Never let anyone tell you "it's all in your head."

2
How Pain Works in the Body

Pain has long been a puzzle to man. But like a jigsaw puzzle, the pieces that explain it are finally being identified one by one and slowly are fitting together to form a big picture.

Pain is a significant event in the body that directly involves all the components of the central nervous system: the brain, the spinal cord, and the acres of nerves. The central nervous system controls the actions of the voluntary muscles, the ones you consciously control. These muscles include the ones you use for walking, waving your hand, or bending your head. Pain also affects the sympathetic nervous system, a component of the autonomic system. The autonomic nervous system controls the involuntary muscles, the ones that you rarely think about. These include the heart muscle that keeps blood pumping, the muscles that open and close (dilate and contract) the diameter of blood vessels, the muscles that contract the pupils in the eyes, and the muscles of respiration that breathe for you without your consciously thinking about it. The sympathetic nerves go to all the arteries in the body, the arteries that control the amount of blood flow to the muscles.

Nerves are a key piece in the pain puzzle. Nerve endings pick up pain messages. Pain messages are started by a stimulus (something that incites action). A pinprick, for example, is a stimulus that starts a pain message. The nerve endings impregnate skin, muscle, bone—almost all the tissue that makes up the human body. Hair, fingernails, and toenails do not have nerve endings, which is why you can cut these parts without feeling pain.

After the never endings pick up a pain message, the message is carried to its final destination by the nerves. Nerves are the pain message conveyor belt, trundling messages to the brain and back to the site where the message began. There are tens of thousands of different nerves throughout the body. The brain alone has billions of nerves and nerve endings. Try to picture nerves as whitish fibers. Some nerves come in bundles, like the bundles of fibers that make up rope, and other nerves may consist of a single strand of material. Some parts of the nerve are coated with a substance called myelin. Myelinated nerves are somewhat like insulated wire; the myelin comes in various thicknesses and acts as an insulator for the electrical charge of the nerve.

All nerves are made up of smaller particles called nerve cells, or neurons. Scientists have been able to photograph cells through a microscope, and they frequently look like irregularly shaped circles.

There are thousands of nerves throughout the body that have been designated by nature as pain nerves. When a stimulus activates a pain nerve's endings, a message of pain travels as an electrical impulse over the nerve fiber from cell to cell along a pathway that takes the impulse to the spinal cord and then on to different parts of the brain. The message travels from cell to cell by a complex series of electrical and chemical processes.

Each nerve cell has transmitter and receiver branches, called axons (transmitters) and dendrites (receivers), that help carry the pain message. The message as an electrical impulse travels from the axons of one cell to the dendrites of a neighboring cell. In order for the message to get to the neighboring cell, it must travel over a gap between the cells. This gap, or junction, is called the synapse. It is at the synapse that the pain message impulse is deciphered and sorted, or "zip coded," so that it travels on in the proper manner. After a message is "zip coded," it might simply move on to the neighboring cell, it might stop at the synapse, or it might be changed at the synapse.

Much has been learned by researchers in recent years about the synapse. The synapse is the center of chemical activity in the nerves, and it is the key for continued transmission of all message impulses.

There are chemical substances associated with the synapse called neurotransmitters (or neurosynaptic transmitters, as they are also known). Neurotransmitters are stimulated into action by the messages carried by the nerve cell. The neurotransmitter is released

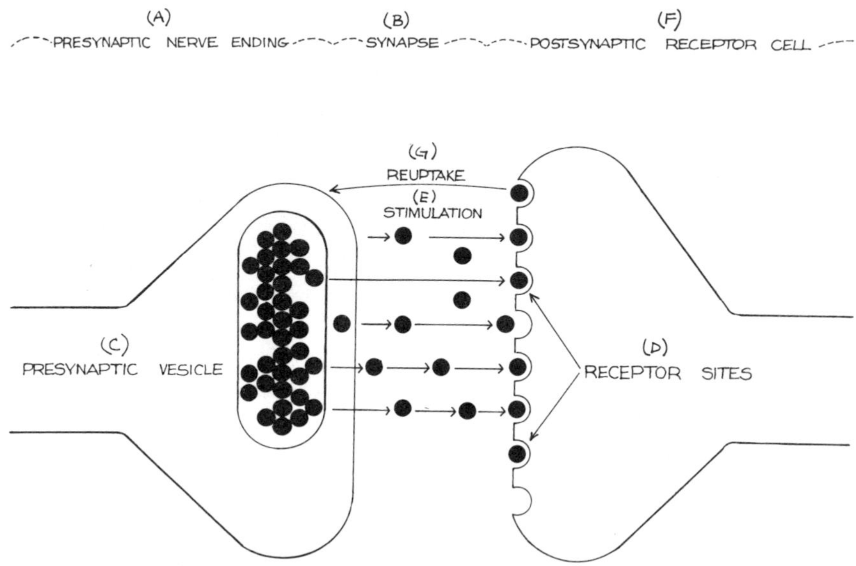

Mechanism of Neurotransmitter Transmission

Neurotransmitters are stored in nerve cells, also called neurons, at the nerve endings (A) near the synapse (B), or the juncture of neighboring cells. The neurotransmitters are stored in storage units called vesicles (C). When an electrical message arrives at a nerve ending (pre-synaptic), the electrical message releases the neurotransmitters stored in the vesicles. A portion of the stored neurotransmitter crosses the synapse carrying the message to the next nerve cell. This transmitted message will be received at the next nerve cell's receptor site (D). This chemical transmission (E) provides specificity, because particular transmitters are found in each nerve: a particular system or pathway may use one type of transmitter, while an adjacent pathway utilizes a completely different chemical.

From "Opiate Receptors and Internal Opiates" by Solomon H. Snyder.

into the synapse from the little vessels that hold the substance within the (pre-synaptic) cell. There, the neurotransmitter chemical acts as a messenger itself—it is the means by which the nerve cells communicate with each other.

When the neurotransmitter chemical is released, it reacts with a receptor, the receiving site of the neighboring (post-synaptic) cell, and conveys or transmits the electrical impulse. You can think of the receptor as a lock and the neurotransmitter as a key. When it turns in the lock properly, everything clicks into place, and the message travels as it was originally intended.

Sometimes the message is changed because of the way the neurotransmitter reacts with the receptor part of the neighboring cell. Things don't click, and the message is changed. In other words, the response of the neighboring cell depends on the ability of its receptor site to recognize and react properly with the neurotransmitter.

Most often, the receptor cell does react appropriately, and the message moves across the synapse and becomes a guided electrical impulse again. The whole process occurs in a fraction of a second and is repeated at each synapse as the message makes its way to its destination.

The transmission process, however, can be reduced (inhibited) or increased (excited), mimicked, or totally blocked—by drugs. A pain message also can be affected by another message traveling along the same nerve pathway, but traveling at a faster speed than the pain message.

Several different chemicals have been identified as neurotransmitters and can be synthesized in a laboratory. These include noradrenaline, also known as norepinephrine, acetylcholine, dopamine, serotonin, and dozens of other less important ones. Different nerve tracts, with their thousands of neurons, contain different neurotransmitters. The different nerve tracts communicate (innervate) the nervous energy, or message, to different parts of the brain.

Recapping: a stimulus activates a pain message in specialized nerve endings. The pain message is transmitted as an electrical impulse from neuron to neuron with the aid of chemicals called neurotransmitters. Neurotransmitters convey the impulse across the synapses that separate cells. The message travels along a pathway to the brain.

Scientists have identified two specific pain pathways to the brain. At first, though, pain messages travel through the spinal cord along a single pathway called the spinothalmic tract. This pathway forks at the brain stem in your neck. One of these branches travels through brain gray matter and the thalamus as well as the hypothalamus (an ancient part of man's brain). This pathway is called the paleospinothalmic pathway, and it is along this one that most dull pain travels. (Interestingly, the majority of chronic pain is described as dull pain, or a variation of dull pain, or throbbing aches.) The paleospinothalmic pathway leads the messages to the limbic system of the brain, the portion of the brain that controls food intake, sexual activity, and the emotions. That the pathway is found here helps to explain why chronic pain has an emotional component.

The other pain-message pathway is called the neo-spinalthalmic pathway, and it conducts sharp localized pain—a good description of most acute pain.

The way pain travels through the spinal cord on its way to the brain is an area of some controversy with pain theorists. A "gate-control" theory was proposed nearly fifteen years ago by researchers Ronald Melzak and Patrick Wall, and its merits are still being debated today.

The gate theory suggests that there is a control mechanism that exists in the "substantia gelatinosa" cells of the spinal cord, a portion of the butterfly-shaped area in the cord. If the gate is open, pain messages will pass through, reach the brain, and make their impact. If the gate is closed, the message will not reach the brain, and, theoretically, you should feel no pain. Melzak and Wall suggest that the "gatekeepers" are nerve-fiber bundles.

According to the theory, small nerve-fiber bundles keep the pathway open, and large bundles, whose signals travel faster than the signals on the small bundles, can close the gate. So the pain of a stubbed toe is transmitted slowly along the small-nerve fibers (designated Delta A and C), and your response of rubbing the painful area stimulates a faster message along the large nerve-fiber bundles (Beta), causing the gate to close and causing you to feel a minimum of pain.

The theory also suggests that the small nerve fibers can multiply the effect of the sensory input to different parts of the brain. Such augmented input, the theorists suggest, would initiate reactive messages from the brain in nerve fibers that descend down through the spinal cord. When enough of these small fibers are activated, a critical threshold is reached in the gate system, a point at which another system is activated by the brain. This is the avoidance system, a reflect phenomenon. It theoretically controls reflex reactions (those performed without thinking) to pain—including the rubbing and scratching you do following the stubbing

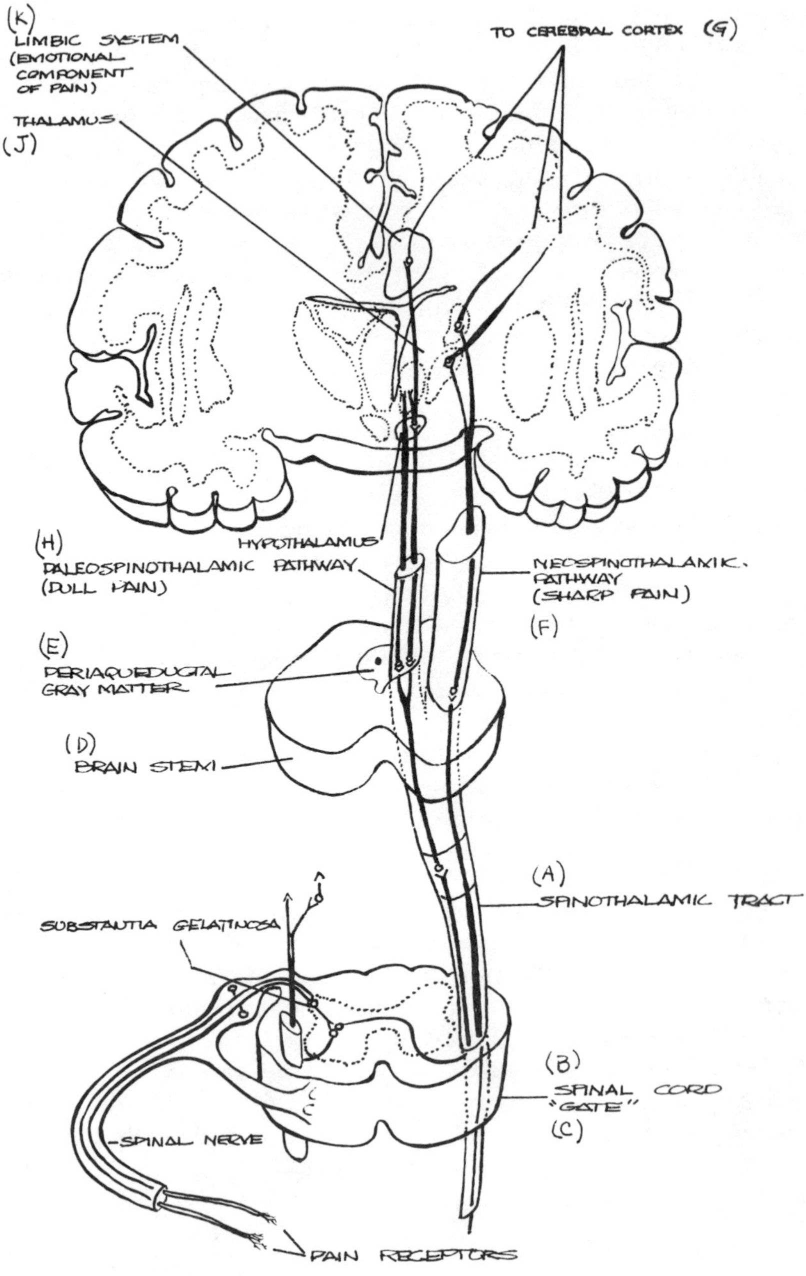
(K)
LIMBIC SYSTEM
(EMOTIONAL
COMPONENT
OF PAIN)
THALAMUS
(J)
TO CEREBRAL CORTEX (G)
HYPOTHALAMUS
(H)
PALEOSPINOTHALAMIC PATHWAY
(DULL PAIN)
NEOSPINOTHALAMIC
PATHWAY
(SHARP PAIN)
(F)
(E)
PERIAQUEDUCTAL
GRAY MATTER
(D)
BRAIN STEM
(A)
SPINOTHALAMIC TRACT
SUBSTANTIA GELATINOSA
(B)
SPINAL CORD
"GATE"
(C)
SPINAL NERVE
PAIN RECEPTORS

of a toe, the swelling and itching that accompanies an insect bite, crying "ouch," or withdrawing a finger or hand from a hot stove. These reactions can be initiated at the spinal cord without any brain (cortical) involvement at all.

While the gate-control theory has yet to be fully accepted by the scientific community, other researchers have gone on to identify an important component of the body's own mechanism for *controlling* pain. In 1977, researchers discovered that bodies internally produced pain killers, endorphins and enkephalins, chemicals similar in molecular structure to potent opiate narcotics such as morphine and heroin. Scientists had theorized since 1973 that chemicals like the endorphins and enkephalins had to exist, because they discovered the brain has many opiate receptor sites. These are sites on cells to which opium and its derivatives, including morphine, heroin, Dilaudid, Talwin, Demerol, Darvon, and Percodan, attach themselves in order to produce their analgesia and euphoric effect. The scientists (notably Snyder, Hughes, and Kosterlitz) reasoned that since such opiates are man-made and are not native to the body—yet there are cells in the body that have a specific affinity for these foreign substances—then the body must produce its own opiatelike substances to attach to the receptor sites.

The opiate receptor sites are located all along the spinal cord

---

Pain Pathways

Pain information travels along two pathways. These pathways receive messages from the dorsal root of the spinal nerve (A), a single pathway that sends messages to the spinal cord (B) in that part of the cord where scientists speculate the pain gateway is located. (The theory suggests that when the gate is open, pain messages pass through to the brain, and when it is closed, the pain messages do not get through.) These impulses go to the spinothalmic tract (C), which branches into two distinct pathways at the brain stem (D). One tract is called the neospinalthalmic pathway (E); it carries mostly acute, or sharp pain messages to the thalamus (F) and cortex (G). The other branch, which travels in the periaqueductal gray matter (H), is called the paleospinalthalmic pathway (I). It carries dull pain messages, such as occur with chronic pain, to the parts of the brain called the hypothalmus (J) and the limbic system (K), ancient portions of the brain that control such human emotions as sex drive and hunger.

From "Opiate Receptors and Internal Opiates" by Solomon H. Snyder.

in the substantia gelatinosa, and they densely populate the paleospinothalmic pathway in the brain. Because this pain pathway goes to the limbic system (which controls emotions), the receptor sites here probably enhance the euphoric effect of the opiates, while the analgesia effect probably begins in the spinal cord.

Scientists have evidence that the endorphins and enkephalins are neurotransmitters, acting at the brain's neuron synapses to influence the integration of sensory information such as pain and emotional behavior.

It is possible that people who seem to feel more pain more often than others may lack endorphins or may have a deficiency of receptor sites. Endorphins someday may also be used as a prescription drug to combat depression and schizophrenia. An increase in endorphins may elevate a person's mood by creating a sense of well-being with an absence of pain everywhere in the body.

The perception of pain, however, is influenced not only by the body's chemical system but by as many as twenty-seven factors identified by Dr. Beecher and other investigators into the mystery of pain.

For instance, experiments have shown that the pain tolerance (the amount of pain a person can tolerate) is lower in different ethnic groups. As part of their heritage and culture, members of certain ethnic groups have "permission" to express pain more freely than another group whose members have been taught to act stoically.

Although physical fatigue seems to have no impact on how much pain a person may feel, mental fatigue does seem to lower the pain threshold in some people (they feel more pain sooner).

The *fear* of pain also lowers the pain threshold. The fear of pain probably works in tandem with anxiety to lower the threshold—if you are anxious about pain occurring, you probably will feel the pain more than if you were not expecting the pain to occur at all. One example of this is getting an injection in a doctor's office. You probably feel the shot in your arm more if you watch as the nurse or doctor gives it to you, than if you are distracted by something going on in the office and don't notice when the shot actually is administered.

The Lamaze method of childbirth is an example of how education about a new process, setting, reduction of anxiety, and the reduction of fear all affect how much pain is perceived. In the

Lamaze-method program, an expectant mother is taught all about the various physical aspects of pregnancy and delivery. Knowing what to expect of and from the body helps to eliminate the fear of the unknown or the anxiety of "what happens next?" The expectant mother also is taught exercises that will help her to cope with the pain and to concentrate on something other than the pain. Many Lamaze-trained women, therefore, are able to go through labor and delivery without analgesics or anesthesia because of their reduced anxiety, reduced tension, distraction from the pain, and an acceptance of the fact that what pain does occur is necessary. This is called "psychoprophylaxis," or preparing the person. The women also know that the pain will end, and that the ending produces a baby.

How you perceive pain can be determined by your family background, your ethnic heritage, and your own personality (see Chapter 4). If, for example, your family believed that it was not proper to complain about pain, you may have a much higher pain threshold than other people. On the other hand, if your family tended to be emotionally expressive and accepted pain as one of life's burdens, you may perceive more pain than others.

Pain, then, is a *subjective* experience that can be explained in part by scientists and only guessed at by others. Some pain can be relieved or, at the least, tempered.

The experience of pain is not confined to any one part of the body, because pain-nerve endings are everywhere (except in the brain itself). Pain can be packaged as a headache that is continuous and incapacitating. Pain can be a chronic sore throat, or a bursitis in your shoulder that seems to get worse when the weather is damp. Your pain can come from the same organic source as your neighbor's pain, yet you may perceive more or less pain and be more or less incapacitated. These individual differences demonstrate the subjective nature of pain perception.

Pain is a message to the spinal cord and brain. You can be conditioned to continue receiving pain messages long after the source of the messages is gone. (Remember Pavlov's dog? The dog was taught to salivate at the sound of a bell because he was always fed soon after a bell was rung.) Pain is a learned pattern, too, and it is rapidly learned because it is, well, painful.

Pain messages can be stopped. They can be stopped by other messages on nerve pathways, or they can be stopped by drugs.

The key thing that differentiates how each individual feels pain is how he perceives it. Think of it this way. There is an old brain twister that asks if a tree falls and no one is near enough to hear it, does the falling tree make a noise when it hits the ground? Applying this to pain perception: if you stub your toe (something that is known to incite pain messages), but your brain is on the blink for some reason (you are on drugs or distracted by something like your house burning down), will you perceive the pain at all?

The answer, of course, is up to the individual, and that is why pain, particularly chronic pain, is so hard to diagnose and treat. While science has discovered many mechanisms and attributes of pain, and how to deal with them, the way individuals perceive pain remains a vast field for theoretical answers. It can't be accurately measured, and that makes the diagnosis and treatment difficult.

Many pieces to the jigsaw puzzle of pain are still missing; many, however, have been discovered, but have yet to be fit into the big picture.

3
Why You Have Chronic Pain:
Some Ailments and Injuries That Can Cause It

Chronic pain is a disease of complex origins and symptoms. It is an indiscriminate enemy. It can originate in the muscles, or begin elsewhere and attack the muscles. It can attack the vascular system, having originated in the venous and arterial systems, or in an entirely different part of the body. It can be neural in origin, emanating from the nerves and the nervous system. Without a doubt, whatever its sources, pain exists on a physical level.

However, there is also an emotional component of human responses that can compound any physical disorder and intensify how much pain any of us perceives. The physical component of pain which often mimics other readily identifiable diseases, can confound the physician when his initial diagnosis is not confirmed by standard diagnostic tests. The emotional component can be a mask, too. Depression, anxiety, fear, and anger can hide underlying physical causes from even the most astute specialist, who is apt to give up and label a chronic-pain sufferer's problem as "psychogenic." Look at the case of a young woman named Jane.

Jane is a woman in her early twenties who had always enjoyed an active, athletic life. About a year ago, just after she graduated from college, she stopped her car at an intersection and a drunken driver slammed into the back of it.

In the emergency room she complained that her neck and left arm hurt her. She was treated and released, but the pain persisted. Her physician, an old family friend, gave her a cervical brace that immobilized her neck in an attempt to alleviate the pain there. When the bracing did not appear to help, another physician, who was called in to consult on the case, put her in traction. Finally she tried denervation (a process during which the nerve is killed by a chemical injected directly into it, or the nerve is severed to kill its effect). This appeared to afford her some relief.

But about eight months after the accident, Jane began to develop pain in her left arm; she felt like pins and needles were pricking her. She went to a neurosurgeon who gave her a thorough work-up and found that the results were all within the limits defined as normal. She went to another neurosurgeon who again found nothing out of the ordinary, no muscles wasting away, no abnormalities on Jane's X-rays. She went to an orthopedic surgeon. He examined all her limbs and could find nothing wrong. He suggested that she see a psychiatrist, claiming the pain apparently was "all in her head."

By the time she arrived at the psychiatrist's office, Jane actually needed her services: she was so deeply depressed that she was close to contemplating suicide. The pain seemed to have taken over her life, and taken the joy out of living. On her doctor's recommendation she checked into an institution for four months of treatment for the depression. However the pain in her left arm persisted after her release, and once again she turned to the psychiatrist for help. Unlike the previous physicians, the psychiatrist listened to her and did not try to talk her out of her pain—when Jane said she had pain, the psychiatrist believed her. This alone gave Jane some measure of relief.

The psychiatrist decided to order a new type of pain-detection test called thermography (see Chapter 6), and the results indicated that the pain was somatogenic (having an organic source) as opposed to psychogenic (having only psychological origins). The physician then tried a drug treatment on her, one that blocks the slower pain-nerve message carriers from reaching the pain receptor sites. The drug therapy was successful. Jane came away from the treatment with a diagnosis (reflex sympathetic dystrophy) that reduced her anxiety, and with significantly less pain—a minimal discomfort that she could bear and that allowed her to go on with her life.

Jane is typical of the legion of chronic-pain sufferers whose disorders somehow fall through the cracks of conventional medical diagnostic systems. While seeking relief, often for many years, these people become afflicted with emotional problems, compounding their perception of pain and perhaps clouding the physician's view of their symptoms and complaints—particularly the physician who is unable or ill-trained to handle severe emotional disturbances.

In Jane's case, the cause of her pain was threefold. The sympathetic dystrophy in her arm (weakening or degeneration of the nerves that innervate the arteries to the arm muscles) was the cause of her left arm pain. Her acute pain was originally caused by the traumas she sustained in her car accident. This physical component then was compounded by her emotional response—her depression at not getting relief, at not finding anyone who believed her complaints, and at the limitations the pain placed on her formally active life. Her emotional state caused her to experience incapacitating pain. These pain cycles that are initiated by trauma and that lead to emotional problems and to increased perception of pain are common in chronic-pain patients.

People who suffer from chronic pain also are liable to increase their troubles through the treatment that they seek. Often their pain is from adhesions (scar tissue attached to healthy tissue inside the body that forms after one or more surgical operations). If the chronic-pain sufferer is taking multiple dosages of different pills prescribed by several physicians, pain can result from the adverse reactions the drugs have on one another and on the body's systems. In some people, if you eliminate the drugs they are swallowing, you may, in fact, completely eliminate the pain. Also, the anxiety of wondering if relief will ever come can heighten the perception of pain.

The following are some of the sources and common causes of chronic pain.

Muscle Pain

Muscular pain probably accounts for more American health complaints than any other source of chronic pain. It is the scourge of millions, who perhaps one morning will wake up and clutch at some point just below the neck and above the buttocks and continue to feel that spot almost every day of their lives.

Back pain can be caused by congenital postural abnormalities, or just bad posture, and by neck injuries, like whiplash; but more often it is linked to degenerative diseases of the intricate muscle and ligament structures in the skeleton that allows humans to walk upright. Dystrophy (weakening or degeneration) and disease often attack the back's muscles and discs, which act as cushions. Should discs slip out of place or become crushed, back pain usually is inevitable.

Low-back pain, located in the small of the back or the axial muscles, is a common complaint. To some degree, this problem is caused by weakened muscles that can be strengthened by exercise. Just being out of shape can open the way for low-back pain. Tension, which can generate muscle spasms, is another source. Low-back-muscle spasms often start with strain or trauma to the region (incorrectly lifting a heavy load can cause such trauma) and then are further aggravated by worrying about the pain, or by any of life's other stresses that accumulate in our daily activities and encounters with other people. These spasms are difficult to diagnose.

Though low-back spasms are common, it is hard for physicians to find evidence that tension and spasms are causing the pain. When you visit your doctor, the spasms may not be present at the exact moment he examines you. If he questions you about your life, you may answer that everything is great, not consciously realizing that you are under any kind of stress or tension, though you actually may be. Once spasmodic low-back pain is diagnosed, however, you will be told that the spasms caused by tension are reversible with the aid of physical therapy (see Chapter 6).

Tension is a stretching or straining of muscles that is often caused by anxiety. This stretching or straining leads to muscular overactivity, producing aches and pains, particularly in the back region. People who often experience a great deal of insecurity, hostility, frustration, and guilt, may also feel anxious and so experience backache.

Sports often lead to *muscle injuries,* and when a certain muscle is injured time after time in the same manner, that muscle may become subject to chronic pain. Knees and ankles are the most likely victims of athletic injuries. These are actually joints not muscles, but when the joint is injured, the ligaments surrounding them may swell and contribute to the pain. Sprains and strains to muscles and joints are easily diagnosed by a trainer, coach, or physician, and treatment usually consists of raising the injured part and packing it with ice. In some cases a tight dressing may be applied to prevent further swelling that could cause hemmorhaging under the skin, and thus additional damage and pain.

Myofascial syndrome is a condition of the body's skeletal muscles. (Myofascial refers to muscles and the cellophanelike membrane that covers the muscles.) It is difficult to diagnose because there is an absence of neurological or orthopedic indicators for it on diagnostic tests. The pain problems associated with myofascial syndrome often mimic conditions such as herniated vertebral discs, syndromes of the joints in the vertebra, pleurisy, and a disease called spondyloisthesis (a displacement of the vertebra producing pain by compression of the nerve root). However, because therapy for this latter group of illnesses is different from therapy for myofascial syndrome, pain relief can be elusive if the diagnosis is incorrect.

Causes of myofascial syndrome include trauma to the neck; muscle tension, such as typists feel in their shoulders after sitting through a long day; and excessive vigorous exercise. In these cases, muscles that normally slide freely against one another are pinned down by adhesions (caused by the trauma). Muscles pulling on the adhesion cause the muscles that are pinned down to go into spasm, since they cannot slide freely.

Physicians can diagnose this syndrome if they can induce pain at several identifiable trigger points in the back. These trigger points are part of muscles and ligaments that, when pressed with a finger, can cause severe pain to radiate outward from the pressure point. The exact etiology (original cause) is as yet not fully understood by physicians, but they speculate that restricting muscle movement produces the initial pain, and this restriction in turn produces a muscle spasm which pulls the sensitive covering over bone to which the muscles is attached, thereby producing more pain.

Another muscular pain is associated with the jaw muscles that control chewing. This syndrome is named after the affected area: the temporomandibular joint, or TMJ. *TMJ syndrome* is a perplexing illness because it, too, mimics the symptoms of more readily identifiable diseases. The symptoms that confound the patient and the physician include pain in the ear, fullness in the ear (as if the ear canal were stuffed with cotton), tinnitus (ringing in the ear), dizziness, or even hearing loss. These signs all appear to be symptoms of a hearing problem, or a problem with one or more of the delicate mechanisms in the ear. A physical examination, however, yields only negative results.

There are several possible causes for TMJ syndrome: one is grinding the teeth, a process often associated with tension that usually occurs while you are sleeping so that you may be unaware that it is happening; another is a dysfunction of one or more of the nerves that ennervate the chewing muscles of the jaw; or a misalignment of the jaw due to natural causes, missing teeth, or trauma. Treatment involves the use of muscle relaxers, anti-inflamation drugs, and EMG biofeedback.

Neural Pain

Trigeminial neuralgia, or *tic douloureux,* is an affliction of a facial nerve (the trigeminial nerve). A bout of neuralgia can be set off by a puff of wind or a slight touch that brushes the face. The pain may disappear within a few hours only to return again, capriciously. Although its cause is as yet unknown, it can be treated (discussed in Chapter 6), using the anti-convulsant drug Tegretol.

Post-herpetic neuralgia is the excruciating aftermath of an adult's bout with herpes zoster, the virus that causes chicken pox in children. The viral infection produces lesions on the skin, similar to chicken-pox marks, but it also leaves lesions under the skin on the nerves of both the central and sympathetic nervous systems. Sometimes when the skin lesions clear up, the lesions on the nerves do not. Large nerve fibers may be destroyed, leaving a greater quantity of the small nerve-fiber bundles—the pain-message conveyors. Therefore, pain messages are sent, and there are no corresponding nerves to countermand them with messages signaling relief. The pain of herpetic neuralgia may be compounded in older people who have atherosclerosis (fatty deposits in the medium and large arteries that restrict the blood flow to parts of the body). Dr. Arthur Taub, at Yale University, has used Elavil and Prolixin to treat this disorder.

Neuromas are tumors that form on nerve endings; they can cause strong and lasting chronic pain. These tumors grow where a nerve has been injured or severed in an accident. Some people are prone to forming neuromas, just as some people are prone to forming keloids, excessive, lumpy-looking scar tissue. No treatment seems truly effective.

Palatal myoclonus is another syndrome found in chronic-pain sufferers. It is a disorder of the palate, the roof of the mouth, in which the muscles in this area expand and contract rapidly, though involuntarily, in a rhythmic (myoclonic) motion. Other muscles in the head and neck may be involved. Palatal myoclonus can be caused by a neurological disorder set off by a trauma, or it can be induced by a vascular disease near the brain stem. Sometimes, physicians are unable to pinpoint the etiology. Sometimes, surgery is effective.

Sympathetic dystrophy is a weakening or degeneration of sympathetic nerves. It is usually caused by trauma to the nerves. Pain associated with sympathetic dystrophy can appear in places that were not affected by the original trauma, as in Jane's case, described earlier in the chapter. Causalgia is a general term used to describe pain caused by nerve damage. It is usually a burning sensation.

Vascular Pain

One of the most familiar forms of vascular pain is the headache, particularly the *migraine headache.* A migraine headache is a throbbing pain caused by spasms of the blood vessels around the brain. These spasms may be brought on by an allergic reaction to some food or substance, though they are frequently the result of frustration, tension, and stress.

Arteries damaged by the buildup of fatty deposits due to *atherosclerosis* also cause chronic pain. The buildup of these fatty deposits can be traced to a high cholesterol diet, or can be the result of an inherited predisposition.

Terminal-Cancer Pain

Terminal-cancer pain is different from most other chronic pain *as there is a definable end for it,* and an easily identified reason for it, whereas with most other chronic pain, the end is unknown.

Terminal-cancer pain is caused by the blockage of organs by tumor growth that has displaced these or other organs from their intended position in the body. The pain can come from the destruction of organs, bones, and other tissue by tumors and from a direct attack by cancer growth on the nerves. Also, radiation, which is sometimes used to treat certain types of cancer, may produce scarring that traps the nerves and produces pain.

Phantom-Limb Pain

Phantom-limb pain is a bizarre manifestation that sometimes follows the amputation of a limb. Patients complain of feeling severe pain in their lost limb. It may be caused by the destruction of nerve endings in the amputated part of the body. Transcutaneous nerve stimulation sometimes helps.

Stomach and Intestinal Pain

Stomachache and *heartburn, pancreatitis, gallstones, chronic constipation, ulcers, ileitis, colitis, polyps,* and *hemorrhoids* are all sources of chronic stomach and intestinal pain. Many of these ailments, including ulcers, heartburn, ileitis, and colitis, are worsened by emotional problems that are translated into stomach pain. Some are degenerative diseases caused by a malfunction of a major organ such as the liver or gallbladder.

Improper diet can result in stomachache. Overdoses of laxatives can produce chronic constipation that causes stomachache. Too much aspirin can bring on gastritis, an irritation of the stomach lining. Overindulgence in alcohol also can lead to gastritis and pancreatitis. Too much coffee or any beverage containing caffeine can contribute to diarrhea and eventually gastritis. Alcoholism can cause an irritation of the stomach lining and subsequent pain. It also can cause pancreatitis and cirrhosis of the liver. Tension and hostility and pent-up anger can aggravate any one of these diseases.

The etiology of ileitis and colitis (painful inflammations of the small and large intestines, respectively) is as yet unknown.

Joint Pain

Arthritis is a disease that afflicts millions and is the most common source of joint pain. It is an inflammation of the joints that attacks hands, fingers, hips—anywhere there are joints in the body. The pain of arthritis can be due directly to the swelling of the joint that exerts pressure on the ligaments and other soft tissues surrounding the joints; pain also results from stiffness due to swelling that limits the use of the joint, which in turn promotes stiffness and pain.

Rheumatoid arthritis is a virulent form of arthritis that causes the soft tissue and skin surrounding the affected joints to thicken into deformities. These changes in the muscles and connective tissues (ligaments) are thought to be caused by deposits of lymphocytes (cells from the lymph glands) thickening the connective tissue. Lymphocytes normally are filtered out of the blood, but this process stops when arthritis sets in.

Gout, once referred to as the rich man's penance for his lifestyle of idleness and excessive food, now is known to be neither the exclusive preserve of the upper classes, nor the result of eating rich food. Gout is a buildup of uric acid in the joints. The acid is manufactured by the kidneys, and when these organs are impaired, they incorrectly process the acid so it is not eliminated as it should be through the urine. This malfunction can be controlled with a drug-therapy regimen and dietary adjustments.

While not exactly a joint disease, *bursitis* feels as if it is attacking the joints. Bursitis is an inflammation of the bursa (any of the fluid-filled sacs that are found surrounding the joints). Bursitis can be caused by a strain or trauma to the bursa or by an infection in the sacs. Housemaid's knee and tennis elbow are popular terms for bursitis in the knee and tendonitis in the elbow.

Headache

Some people are plagued with chronic headaches. Not all headaches are located in the same part of the head, nor do they occur for the same reasons. Muscle tension headaches, which account for 90% of all headaches, are caused by tension, annoyance, or other repressed feelings that lead to muscle spasms. These are usually felt in the back of the head. Eyestrain from overwork, improper prescriptions for glasses, or the need for corrective lenses can also push the muscles around the eyes into spasm. This headache may be felt in the eyes or around the temple area.

The *ice-cream headache* is associated with a cooling of a blood vessel in the palate, due to ingesting any very cold food or drink. As the arteries cool, they constrict and cut off the flow of blood to the skin or sinuses or ophthalmic arteries, causing pain. Avoid eating ice cream too quickly or gulping iced drinks, and you can avoid the ice-cream headache. Rubbing your tongue against your palate rapidly relieves this headache.

Cluster headaches attack in several areas at once, sometimes grouping around the temple on one side of the head. These headaches are thought to be an allergic reaction as histamine is found in the tissue cells on the affected side. Histamine (a substance that causes capillaries and veins to dilate) is released when there is an injury to the skin or membranes, such as a reaction by the membranes to an allergin. Recent articles suggest lithium may be a useful treatment.

Migrain headaches are usually described as excruciating. They, too, are thought to be an allergic reaction. Doctors believe migraines to be an allergy because they can bring on an attack with the injection of histamine into a migrain-sensitive person. Acute migraines can be accompanied by nausea and double vision in addition to the pain, described as high-intensity throbbing. However, at least fifty different etiologies have been described.

Another source of chronic headaches frequently overlooked by physicians, are head pains caused by trauma to muscles nowhere near the head—for example, muscles in the shoulder, face, back, and neck. These muscles can be irritated by bad posture, eyestrain, a short leg, the results of surgical procedures on the neck or the excessive use of neck muscles for respiration in a person who suffers from chronic obstructive lung disease.

What causes chronic pain? As you can see, any number of factors beyond your control: overuse of muscles, accidents, genetic predisposition, viruses, middle and old age, and emotions that you don't even know you are experiencing. Whether chronic pain is brought on by some outside agent, such as a car accident resulting in a case of whiplash, or some internal disorder, a breakdown of the organs in your body, how you handle the pain, how you accept it and regard it, plays an important role in the frequency and the intensity of what you feel.

4
Copers, Mopers, Exaggerators, and Malingerers:
Pain and Personality

Has anyone you know ever said something like "the pain in this tooth is going to drive me crazy" or "it's hardly worth getting out of bed in the morning, my back hurts so much"? Many people have had occasion to voice these sentiments. Whether it is in the form of a backache that doesn't go away or a headache that becomes a part of your life, chronic pain is an unwanted houseguest—it is a disrupter of your daily routine, the habits that make you feel secure or content with life. Such an intruder constantly demands attention, so that there is no time left for yourself, there is only time for your unwanted guest. It steals all your energy and becomes the focus of your life. Because of its intrusive nature and demand for attention, chronic pain can change your life, can change the way you behave and the way you feel. In other words, pain affects your personality—the sum total of your physical, emotional, and social characteristics—and your personality, in turn, determines the changes pain, chronic pain, effects in you.

The following is a case history that describes how pain and personality affect each other.

Martha is a middle-aged housewife who was happy with her life. Turning fifty didn't phase her; growing older just meant there was more breathing space for her. Her children, who had been difficult adolescents, were finally grown up, decently she thought, and they had all left the nest to make their own way. She was confident that she had done her best by them.

Martha's husband had recently achieved seniority in his union, so their financial future was looking good, and with the children gone, she finally had some time to herself. She kept the house the way she wanted to and she got herself a part-time job in the local hardware store, run by her cousin.

One day while discussing a sale with her cousin, she noticed that her voice sounded different, as if she had a frog in her throat. Her cousin mentioned something to that effect, too. Over the next few days her voice did not get better, so she thought she was coming down with laryngitis. She took to her bed and dosed herself with aspirin and cold-medicine time capsules. But her voice did not get better. Reluctantly, she went to see the family doctor, who, after examining her throat, referred her to an ear, nose, and throat specialist, an otolaryngologist. This doctor told Martha that one of the vocal cords in her throat was palsied (shaking) because of a degenerating muscle. Surgery would have to be performed if her voice were to sound the same again.

Martha was afraid to have the operation. She did not particularly like doctors, and she definitely did not like hospitals. In fact, she had never had surgery. But she knew she had to have the surgery. Her husband told her the sound of her voice was disconcerting, and at times that he was annoyed by it because he did not recognize it. After thirty years, he was used to hearing her speak in a certain way. Additionally, the customers at the store were complaining that they couldn't understand her. So, in order to get her life back to normal, Martha consented to the operation.

The otolaryngologist explained that the surgery was a fairly complicated procedure: it involved making an incision just above her collarbone and attaching one of her good vocal muscles to the weakened one. The idea of the incision terrified her; she told him it sounded as if he were going to cut her throat. Despite her fears, she consented to the procedure and the operation was a success.

After her recovery, Martha's voice sounded fine—just the way it used to sound. But now she complained that her left arm felt numb and hurt, a burning sensation. How could an operation on her throat have side effects like that, she wondered—and so did the specialist. He told her family doctor that he thought her complaint was a hysterical conversion, that she had converted her fear and anxiety about the operation into pain in order to continue receiving the extra attention she had received while hospitalized. Both doctors told her to ignore the pain.

Martha could not ignore the pain. It was always there. If she tried to do housework, it felt worse. If she was working in the hardware store, she got distracted from what she was doing and gave out the wrong change or no change at all. She complained to her husband, and he complained back to her. He wanted her to stop griping.

But how could she stop griping. She seemed to hurt all the time. She hated hurting, and she resented the constant pain. She kept asking herself "Why me?" "What did I do to deserve this pain?" Then she felt sorry for herself and hurt all the more. She cursed the pain, cursed her husband who did not seem to understand, and ended up cursing herself for having the operation that left her with the pain.

She tried to adjust to the pain, after she finished cursing it. She appeared to vascillate more and more between hate and acceptance. She stopped keeping an immaculate house. All that bending, stretching, lugging, walking, and polishing did not seem to be worth the effort. She did, however, keep the house well enough so that her husband would not notice the difference. She was scared that he might be even more angry with her, aside from her complaints of pain, if she stopped doing the one thing she thought she did best.

She quit her job, though, because her cousin didn't understand her anymore, did not want to gossip with her over coffee, did not want to pal around with her in general because, her cousin said, the topic was always the pain in Martha's arm. Martha had become a complaining nag.

Martha once more went to her physician, and he prescribed some pain killers; but as soon as they wore off, she was aware of the pain again. She became bitter and depressed about not having a job anymore, and she was angry at her husband. She was no longer a contented person and did not look forward to doing anything.

Martha eventually went to another physician who took a series of tests. Most of the tests were negative—the only thing that seemed to be wrong was that the scar on her left collarbone was hypersensitive to touch. Her left arm and hand retained a normal appearance. Thermography, however, turned up a mild reflex sympathetic dystrophy. Some of the nerves controlling the blood vessels to Martha's left arm and hand had been slightly damaged during her first operation. The physician performed several sympathetic nerve blocks (an injection of a chemical into a sympathetic nerve in order to kill the nerve), and this gave Martha quite a bit of relief. Physical therapy also was prescribed. With the bending and stretching exercises, the pain lessened even more.

Martha returned to work and does as she pleases once again. She's not as happy as she once was, though. She retains some bitterness for her husband and cousin who did not believe her when she was in constant pain.

Martha's pain changed her from a fairly happy woman with a bright outlook on life and a good relationship with her husband and friends to a depressed person no one wanted to associate with—and she didn't care. Pain had become the focus of her life.*

* Based on material from Chapter 104 by Nelson H. Hendler, in Youman's *Textbook of Neurosurgery,* Saunders, Philadelphia, 1979.

Not all chronic-pain patients adjust or react to pain in the same manner as Martha. How a person adjusts to daily, intractable pain in part is determined by his "premorbid" adjustment. Premorbid refers to the time before the person became afflicted with pain; his adjustment refers to a description of what he was like, what kind of relationships with other people he maintained, and how he felt about himself, before the pain began.

To better understand how pain and personality interact, chronic-pain patients can be categorized, very generally, into four types. These categories are also useful to physicians in deciding a course of treatment. The categories divide the different patient personalities along lines of comparison, for instance, comparing a patient's premorbid adjustment to his adjustment to life with pain.

Another factor that differentiates chronic-pain patients is the "chronicity" of pain—how long has the patient actually experienced the pain, how much of his life has the pain taken over, and what activities did focusing on pain replace?

Onset of pain is still another important element in the development of a chronic-pain-personality type. For example, was the pain originally due to an injury or a physical trauma, or did it appear out of nowhere one day? Is the pain located in a specific area or is it located in a general area that is difficult for the patient to pinpoint?

The environment or day-to-day circumstances beyond a person's control also will affect how he handles pain. Pain may be more evident to someone who has a healthy spouse to depend on, or it may be less evident, perhaps pushed into the background, by the spouse who is needed for a family's support and places this responsibility above the pain and refuses to allow the pain to interfere.

Money often plays a large role in the life of a person who is in pain. The availability of workmen's compensation, social security disability payments, and unemployment insurance can determine how you handle pain and, in many cases, can affect your recovery.

Using factors like those listed above, we have categorized chronic-pain patients as: Type I, the Copers; Type II, the Exaggerators; Type III, the Mopers; and Type IV, the Malingerers (conscious and unconscious). These categorizations were based on observations of working with nearly 2,000 chronic-pain patients over five years. They are generalizations—some people have some traits that are appropriate to more than one category. They are meant to serve only as a framework to help you better understand how personality can affect pain and how pain can mold personality.

Type I, the Copers

About half of the chronic-pain patients probably fall into the coper category. The coper is a stable person who at one time felt his life was well-organized and who suddenly becomes afflicted with a condition about which he knows nothing. He tries to cope with it, with this chronic pain, but fails. He then is unable to keep his life on an even keel while fighting the pain.

In most copers seen at the Johns Hopkins pain clinic, the pain could be directly traced to a lesion or some problem that showed up on diagnostic tests. When asked about their lives before the pain, they were described by the patients as "normal"—married, a decent work record, and a tendency to follow a fairly regular routine: work, homelife, sleep, and work. But chronic pain interrupted the pattern, and interrupted it negatively.

When the pain lasts between two weeks and two months, the coper acts as if nothing is wrong; he takes the pain in his stride. He may even try to "beat" it by speeding up his activity, usually against the recommendation of his physician. He will return to work earlier than was recommended.

He will try to ignore the pain, sluff it off as something temporary, refuse to recognize that the pain is causing him any disability, and will not allow his friends or family to sympathize with him. Pain to the coper is just one of life's pitfalls. It is encountered, then conquered. Basically, he denies the problem.

However, if the pain lasts as long as six months, it begins to take its toll on this normally stable personality. The coper becomes touchy and angers easily. He has difficulty falling asleep and sometimes even is awakened from sleep by the pain. He begins to take pain-killers, when formerly he rarely would put an aspirin in his mouth. His life becomes a little more lonely, he doesn't go out as often as he used to, and he doesn't try to socialize with people at work during coffee breaks or other free times.

When the pain becomes entrenched, when it claims from six

months to eight years of his life, the coper inevitably becomes depressed. This kind of depression is not a "down in the dumps" or a temporary "blue" feeling. This depression is a serious illness, not just a health hazard but a hazard to life. He is depressed because he feels he has lost something—lost the ability to be his former self. This once stable person now begins to think of suicide as a method of escaping pain. He has lost hope that the pain ever will go away and has refashioned his life around the realization. He may have altered his work habits to accommodate his pain (such as a warehouseman not lifting heavy items), or he may have quit working altogether. Depression, in fact, is a common accompaniment to chronic pain, no matter what the personality type.

Depression is not the only emotional response of the coper, after years of enduring the pain. His emotional expression may run the gamut from anger (a "why me?" attitude) to despair. The coper may attempt to bargain with his doctor(s)—he now tells him that he doesn't care if all the pain is eliminated; he will settle for the relief of some of it, although he knows in advance that his request will not be fulfilled.

All these stressful emotions are affecting his relationships with other people. His marriage now is not as happy as it once was, and his sexual activity is kept to a minimum, if there is sex at all. There is a great deal of self-pity expressed to family and friends, and the coper begins to think of himself as an albatross around everyone's neck: he's no fun to be with anymore, so he decides that maybe it's best if he keeps to himself.

Pills as well as pain have become the focus of his life. His habitual use of narcotics has led, as it so often does, to addiction: the coper thinks that if one pill is good, then two are certainly better, and so on until he is unable to function without the pills.

Betty Ford, wife of ex-President Gerald Ford, is a good example of a typical coper. In the spring of 1978, Mrs. Ford publicly and frankly admitted that she was addicted to pain killers and alcohol. Her previous bouts with bad health were already well known. While her husband was President she underwent a mastectomy for breast cancer. She also suffered from osteoarthritis (a form of arthritis that attacks the bones) that affected her back, and in addition was plagued by a pinched nerve in her neck. She told the press that her neck and back had bothered her for more than ten years.

When she talked to the public again in 1978 about her health, she said that she was checking into a California hospital to be detoxified, to overcome her addiction to medications and alcohol. She issued a statement to the public stating that drug dependence "is an insidious thing and I mean to rid myself of its damaging effects."

Betty Ford coped with her pain for more than ten years in the best way she knew how. She continued to work and to contribute to her husband's campaign, all the time sustaining this activity with the coper's last resort—pain pills. But because she wanted to restore the life she used to live, she had herself detoxified.

Getting on with life as it was—that's the key to the coper personality.

The coper lives with pain, but never really believes that he will have to do so for the rest of his life, so he does not allow the pain to completely disable him—he retains some measure of control over his life. He is depressed, but he goes on.

After years of having pain as a "roommate" in his body, he adjusts and adjusts well. He may give up narcotics, and find that he can sleep as easily as when he was pain-free. He readjusts his goals. This is the single, most critical adaptive mechanism for a chronic-pain patient, since pre-pain expectations of achievement are unattainable. If these goals are maintained, then he constantly feels like a failure. However, if he acknowledges his limitations, and readjusts his life situations to suit new, perhaps lesser expectations, he again enters the world of reality, not wishful thinking, and can better accept himself as a "functioning" human being—not a "cripple."

A primary treatment goal for the Type I chronic-pain patient should be the reduction of his anxiety about his pain. By reducing the anxiety, it becomes less likely that his work, sleep, eating, and sex habits will be affected. By fighting anxiety, the physician also helps the coper to ward off tension and prevent possible resulting muscle spasms that can create more pain. If surgery seems to be called for, it probably should be done, as the coper has a good prognosis for recovery and adjustment following such procedures—better than any of the other categories of chronic-pain patients.

Martha, who was described at the beginning of this chapter, is a good example of a Type I chronic-pain personality, a coper. Martha was well-adjusted before her pain began. Her reaction was to cope, and with the aid and support of a physician who understood her problem, she was able to return to the life she had left behind while she was concentrating on her pain.

Type II, the Exaggerators

Joan is an example of another category of pain patient—the exaggerator. Joan is younger than Martha, somewhere in her mid-thirties. Joan never was as happy as she wanted to be nor did she ever have enough of what she thought she deserved. Joan dropped out of high school and married a mechanic, more because she wanted to get away from her parents than because she loved him. Joan stuck with her husband through a few joyless years until she could not stand him or his friends any longer. She divorced him and never saw him again.

Joan went home to her parents and was miserably unhappy. She drifted in and out of reality with the help of her parents' liquor supply. If she did not like what was happening during the day—if her mother criticized her for being sloppy—she turned to alcohol for comfort. She decided to do something spectacular before her twentieth birthday: she would kill herself. She thought the easiest way would be to drink herself into happy oblivion and then swallow all the sleeping pills she could find. Her parents, however, discovered her before she could take too many pills and rushed her to an emergency room where they pumped her stomach and saved her life.

Joan went back to her parents' house to live. Instead of raiding their liquor cabinet, though, she started going down to the neighborhood singles' bar, where she met her second husband. When they first started dating, he told her he wanted to make the Army his career; after asking Joan to marry him, he enlisted. This did not thrill her, but he was sent to Vietnam before she really decided to protest his decision. While he was gone she discovered she was pregnant and decided that she had to go live with her parents again, since she could not take care of a baby alone.

Her husband returned after two years in combat, without a scratch and with an officer's commission. The officer's larger paycheck gave Joan some pleasure. Joan and her husband and child moved on to the Army base in her hometown, where her husband insisted they raise the family.

In order to get a promotion, after several year's of peace-time duty, Joan's husband thought he would have to find a job in the Army that would let him travel and show his superiors what he could do. Joan protested, especially since she was pregnant with their second child. She had not liked raising one child alone while he was overseas, and the thought of dealing with two alone absolutely terrified her.

He started traveling anyway. While he was gone Joan got a prescription from a base doctor for Valium to calm her nerves. With two young preschool children screaming all day, she started getting horrible headaches, and her doctor gave her a prescription for Percodan, a narcotic.

After several years of traveling, her husband decided to make his career as a teaching supervisor permanent, and Joan learned that she would be alone eight months of every year. This did not help her headaches. In fact, her headaches started disturbing her sleep. Once more she went to a base doctor, and this time he prescribed Seconal, a barbiturate-type sleeping pill.

Despite all the pills, and even with the first child in school, Joan's headaches continued. By the time her oldest was in second grade the pain seemed to be continuous and no longer confined to headaches; now she was also bothered by pain around her eyes and cheeks. She decided that the base doctors hadn't helped her in the last few years (all they did was renew her prescriptions for Valium, Seconal, and Percodan), so she went off the base to see another physician. This third physician prescribed a more potent narcotic for her and told her to come back in a few weeks if the pain was not gone. A few weeks later, however, she was in another state visiting her husband.

While she was there she saw another doctor who prescribed something for the pain and something to help her sleep at night—Joan had not told her that she already was taking Seconal. At the suggestion of her husband, Joan went to see yet another doctor who specialized in the treatment of eye ailments (an ophthalmologist). Perhaps, her husband said, the headaches and eye pain were attacking her because she needed glasses. The eye doctor could find nothing wrong.

By now, the pain after seven years of almost constant headaches, was making her vomit daily, and she was dizzy most of the time. She could no longer get out of bed in the morning. The pain, she said, was keeping her in bed and driving her to distraction. Sometimes it was so bad that she did not bother to get out of bed at all. Her husband came home from one of his long trips and found her in bed crying pitifully from the pain. He called the base doctor, who decided it was time to hospitalize her.

After two weeks the staff physicians said they could find nothing, yet Joan still complained of severe headaches and sharp throbbing pains behind her eyes. She told the hospital physicians that she also had pain in her shoulders, particularly when she woke up in the morning. After a few more weeks of running tests, the doctors said that there was nothing more that they could do for Joan. They wanted to discharge her. Joan said that although she missed her wonderful husband and children, she did not want to leave the hospital. The pain scared her. She had had it for so long she did not think that she could trust herself to be alone—she was desperate. She was thinking about suicide again, just to end the pain, because she knew that it could only get worse.

The exaggerator has two basic traits: he has a poor pre-pain adjustment and his complaints that the pain interferes with his life are in excess of what one might expect from his problem.

A poor premorbid adjustment in the exaggerator can be tied to a variety of factors: organic brain disease, anxiety neuroses, obsessive-compulsive personality, paranoid-schizophrenic personality, dependent personality, hysteric personality, Briquet's syndrome, and psychosomatic problems.

The organic brain diseases that contribute to poor pre-pain adjustment include such conditions as senility (from hardening of the arteries due to old age or disease) and drug-induced dementia (aberrant behavior) that often is concommitant with prolonged alcoholism or drug abuse or mixing the two substances. Pain is exaggerated by these conditions and seems to be more debilitating than it probably is.

The exaggerator with organic brain disease will complain to his doctor that he has trouble remembering things, can't concentrate, and can't seem to think on his feet as well as he used to. His family will report that he is more irritable and has trouble sleeping. He will then say that all problems are due to and started with the onset of his pain. Although tests will show that it has some organic source, the pain seems to be greater than what such physical injuries or traumas usually should produce. Diagnosis of organic brain disease can be made at the same time that the sources of the pain are being investigated by an electroencephalogram (an EEG, a brain-wave chart) or by X-ray scanning of the brain (a CAT scan).

Treatment for this patient usually consists of drugs and supportive psychotherapy for the family. With the diagnosis, other forms of treatment seem to fall in place. Once the family knows what is wrong with the exaggerator, they have fewer expectations of his performance. If the patient understands the problem he places less pressure on himself to perform and has less anxiety about what is wrong with him. He therefore has less need to exaggerate his pain and his complaints will diminish. What happens in these cases is that the patient is so relieved to find out what is wrong, that his diminished capacities are due to an organic rather than psychological cause, that he experiences relief of anxiety and copes better with whatever discomfort exists, rather than relying on and even exaggerating the pain to excuse those frightening changes in his abilities.

Another exaggerator is Corinne, a fifty-six-year-old widow who lost her husband about five years ago.

About two years into her widowhood, when she was feeling particularly lonely, she began to experience low-back pain, and pain in her leg, neck, and shoulder. Corinne was always a complainer—nothing ever really had satisfied her in her adult life. She had been married twice before she married Joe, who died of a bleeding ulcer only two years after they were married.

Three years after the pain began, Corinne told her family physician that it was getting worse. He treated her with facet blocks (an injection of a numbing agent directly into the back joints) in her back and she reported that she had experienced some relief. But she soon was back in his office complaining that now she had pain in her shoulder, neck, and one arm. Her physician took some X-rays, but they did not show anything wrong in these areas. This time he performed some denervations, and Corinne told him that she felt some relief in her neck, shoulder, and arm; however, these pains were replaced with pain in her lower back and leg, and she had headaches near her forehead.

Next her physician took an electroencephalogram, and an IQ test, as he suspected that she might be suffering from organic brain disease. There were some abnormalities on both the tests, so he questioned Corinne more closely about her personal life and medical history during the past year.

After her husband died, Corinne had started working as an insurance agent, which provided an outlet for her frustrations by occupying her time as well as giving her some satisfaction—she was making her own money for the first time in her life. However, since her pain began three years before, she had not been as active in getting new clients as she thought she should be. This worried her. After the operation she began to have difficulty with her concentration and memory—just about the same time the pain became debilitating. She felt that her business was now in great jeopardy because the pain made it uncomfortable for her to sit for a long time in a car, and this made driving the long distances her job demanded almost impossible.

During the pain period, Corinne greatly reduced her activity at work. She also became depressed about her reduced concentration, memory impairment, and general condition. She was angry and upset that a younger agent was allowed to service her new accounts, and her boss set her to work at the mundane job of typing up reports.

With the information about her impaired memory and loss of concentration powers, and the results of the EEG and IQ tests, her doctor made a diagnosis of early organic brain disease, which he broke to Corrine as gently as possible. At first disturbed by the news, Corinne claimed that later she felt greatly relieved. She thought that the reduction in her abilities to think on the job was due to emotional illness, and she actually felt better knowing that it was a physical problem.

Her physician prescribed low doses of a mood elevator and suggested that she return to work, not as a high-powered front-running agent, but as an office worker. The lowered expectations that she had for herself and the lowered expectations that her boss had for her, once he learned of the diagnosis, helped her to cope with the residual pain that she felt. But the pain was no longer described as incapacitating.

Another type of patient who exaggerates his pain is the person who premorbidly is afflicted with anxiety or depression neuroses (an emotional disorder in which anxious or depressing thoughts dominate the personality). These neuroses may have been brought on by the death of a close relative, divorce, problems with children, financial difficulties, or problems with sex. Stressful situations like these that result in a loss, whether it is the loss of a person or possession, can result in depression. Psychiatrists agree that it is hard to separate anxiety from depression and that generally a depressed person is also anxious. The reaction of this type of person to pain will be immediate as well as exaggerated.

There may actually be a lesion or some form of arthritic change that shows up on an X-ray. But the exaggerator with anxiety neuroses will cease functioning much more quickly than the coper. He will start abusing drugs sooner, gain weight almost immediately because of inactivity, and readily complain about anxiety and pain.

A careful history of this Type II patient's premorbid adjustment will help to delineate his problems and differentiate him from the coper. The key to diagnosis is the immediacy of the patient's response after the onset of pain and an overconcern about the pain. Treatment for pain that in part can be attributed to a lesion or trauma can include denervations or blocks.

The outcome for this exaggerator can be bright if the source of the anxiety and depression can be identified. Medication may be effective, but the best therapy for this type of patient is psychotherapy. This can help him to cope with the pain by helping him to understand not only the conflicts in his life that contribute to his depression but how his depression contributes to his perception of pain.

People who are afflicted with anxiety and depression can come from all walks of life.

Peter, a fortyish attorney married to an attorney who works in the same firm, is a good example of an exaggerator who has a generalized anxiety that contributes to his increased perception of and complaints about pain.

Four years ago Peter fell down while walking to work and ruptured a disc in his back; he had the disc removed. Although the pain had stopped for a time following the operation, it returned and for three years bothered not his back but rather his shoulder, right arm, and neck. Most of the neurological tests he underwent were normal, but one X-ray revealed that he had degenerative osteoarthritis (an arthritis of the bone that gets progressively worse) in his neck.

His physician performed several denervations in the neck area. During the time he was hospitalized for these operations, Peter had several long talks with his doctor. The doctor noticed that he was depressed. His color was bad, he had dark circles under his eyes, he had a perpetual frown, and his conversation was rarely lightened with laughter. Peter admitted one day that the pain was making him depressed and worried him because he felt that it was causing trouble for him at work. The pain made it difficult for him to write.

Because Peter also said he was having difficulty sleeping at night, the doctor prescribed a mood elevator to help him deal with the depression anxiety and to help him fall asleep.

Peter also entered psychotherapy. During that time, he learned that his wife was carrying on a flagrant affair with a colleague. At first he had refused to believe that she was having an affair, but finally was forced to accept it when he opened some of her letters to her lover.

Since he worked with his wife, he thought that she should quit and leave the firm so he wouldn't have to be confronted with her infidelity on a daily basis. She did not quit, and his pain got progressively worse. At the same time his sexual activity decreased to about once a month. He claimed that by not having sex he avoided some measure of pain.

After another year of therapy, Peter finally confronted his wife about her affair and about how intolerable he felt their work situation was. She agreed to end her extramarital relationship and enter therapy with Peter. After six months of joint therapy with his wife, Peter found that his pain was no longer unbearable, merely uncomfortable.

Peter admitted that it was while he was under stress at home and at work that he felt most depressed. When he was most depressed, his pain became more than he could tolerate. With his new relationship with his wife and some understanding about himself, Peter now could cope with the pain.

Another Type II pain patient prone to exaggeration has an obsessive-compulsive personality, and this trait contributes to his poor premorbid adjustment.

This exaggerator is an inhibited and rigid person; he is overwhelmingly preoccupied and concerned with living by the rules and standards and traditions he has known since childhood. He is conservative and dogmatic in his thinking, meticulously neat, and opinionated. Decision-making is almost impossible for him, as every possibility must be evaluated and thoroughly examined in advance.

Perfection is his hallmark. He is attracted to jobs that are precise in nature, such as tool and die making, which is repetitive, watchmaking, computer programming, or neurosurgery—all exacting professions for details. This type of pain patient is usually a steady worker with no financial difficulties or marital strife.

Because pain upsets the perfect harmony in his life, this patient views pain that impairs his control or disables him as simply intolerable and unbearable. Even minor injuries will affect him to an unusual degree. Though not a hypochondriac, he is similar to one in his overconcern about the threat of pain and injury. His pain usually has an organic basis. Pain will disrupt his sleep schedule by hampering his ability to get to sleep, and his sexual activity will be reduced because of the pain. But this patient will adhere to whatever the doctor orders for his cure of relief.

This exaggerator can be diagnosed with standard diagnostic tests and treated with mood-elevating drugs or with surgery. He wants to be cured and will follow whatever is recommended. With assurance from the family doctor or surgeon about his recovery, this patient should improve and his complaints of pain will diminish

Herb, a forty-year-old mechanic, is a native of West Germany. He is the product of a strict religious household and the son of a mother who was obsessively neat. He came to the United States about twenty years ago, mostly to escape from the confines of his family and his background.

Three years ago Herb woke up with a pain in his lower back. He had spent most of the evening before working on an old car for a good customer. The engine just did not sound right to him; and he had tinkered with it for hours until it had made the sounds he wanted to hear. The customer had been calling him hourly, overanxious about the old vehicle, and this had made Herb even more determined to do a perfect job. When he went home, he kept thinking about the car, wondering if he actually had done as good a job as he could, and slept poorly. The next morning he woke up with the pain.

The pain persisted for several months. Depending on the weather and how much work he put in during a day, it could feel either sharp or dull; in either case it seemed to worsen in damp weather. Sometimes the pain shot down his right leg, and this hampered his bending motion and made him furious that he couldn't look at his engines as closely as he thought he should.

All the tests his doctor ordered were within the normal limits, but Herb continued to complain that the pain was interfering with his sleep and his concentration. He also said that it was getting in the way of his work and sex life. He said that what he feared most was that it could lead to permanent disability, or maybe even to a bedridden life. It took months before he shared this fear with his doctor, and when he finally did, he added that should he become permanently disabled he was afraid that he would have to return to his parents' home for them to care for him.

Herb's physician prescribed a mood elevator; the pills helped him to sleep at night and relax during the day. He also prescribed electrical stimulation to the affected area (see Chapter 6). As the relief Herb received increased, so did his confidence about his future, and some of his fears about being permanently bedridden disappeared. Finally, his physician felt he was ready for a denervation (the killing of a nerve); this gave him the best relief yet.

However, one source of anxiety remained. Although most of his discomfort was gone, and he had to admit to himself that what was left of it was bearable, he continued to worry about what was causing the pain. He was afraid that any day it could return, in a more violent form, and never go away.

After repeated assurance from his neurosurgeon and a three-week stay at a pain-treatment center where he learned to relax with biofeedback ** and began to rid himself of some of his anxiety about being disabled, Herb stopped worrying about his pain. Without the worry he concentrated better, and went back to work, focusing his attention on mechanics rather than on his pain.

The Type II personality who is a paranoid or paranoid schizophrenic usually has a history of psychiatric hospitalizations. This person probably is single or divorced or has been separated many times from a spouse and his work record is similar to his marital track record—many job changes, a poor level of performance, extended absenteeism. He may also have a history of drug abuse and may have been jailed several times for drug problems or even for assault.

Because this type of personality has difficulty perceiving reality correctly, he may view his pain as an attack by hostile forces outside his body. He exaggerates the pain as he exaggerates other situations.

The pain may be the result of an injury or it may have come on slowly. If hospitalized for the pain, this exaggerator will be a somewhat hostile patient, guarded and belligerent, demanding instant service from the nurses and immediate relief from the doctors. This patient can be diagnosed through psychiatric tests and a history obtained from the family.

Drug treatment usually can reduce the complaints of pain, and with psychiatric care this patient can return to work or return home as a functioning member of the household.

Neal, an unmarried young man who works in a warehouse, is a good example of this type of exaggerator. He injured his lower back in the winter of 1973 when lifting a box that was heavier than he thought. Immediately he felt a pain in his back, and by the next morning he also had a pain in his right leg. The company doctor could find nothing wrong but decided to refer him to a neurologist. The neurological examination showed that everything was functioning within normal limits.

** Biofeedback is a new treatment method that measures either muscle tension or temperature of a person's back or limbs and makes him aware of this physical phenomenon. He can then use this awareness to help modify the causes of his pain.

After several years of pain in his back and leg and after visiting a dozen doctors, Neal was furious—all the time. He had seen a neurosurgeon soon after his injury and now decided to go back to him. This time he demanded that he be cured and threatened that if he were not, the neurosurgeon might not live to treat another patient.

The doctor remained calm and had a long talk with his patient, after which Neal decided to trust him, to take him into his confidence. He told the physician that there were people at work who were jealous of him and who were putting poison into his food. The poison was causing the back pain. The neurosurgeon then referred Neal to a psychiatrist, who treated him and placed him on a potent tranquilizer, Thorazine.

Neal still complains of back pain from time to time, but he has been able to return to work.

The dependent personality is similar to the exaggerator who has some sort of anxiety or depressive neuroses. This person's poor premorbid adjustment is characterized, however, not by depression or stress but by an unhealthy inability to live independently of others.

A person of this type may have had a long-standing reliance on a parent for emotional support and may still maintain frequent and intimate contact with the parent. On the other hand, he may have been rejected or abandoned as a child and have become dependent on others because of this rejection.

If he works, this individual probably holds a position in a protected job He is probably a passive person, outwardly compliant, and has not achieved a high degree of success as a result of his fear of conflict.

When struck with pain, this person immediately becomes attached to a doctor and is eager and willing to comply with all the orders and prescription instructions he receives. He may become addicted to Valium or narcotics and will be moderately or severely incapacitated by the pain. He will complain loudly and frequently about the pain and may gain twenty pounds from inactivity.

It is hard to diagnose this type of pain patient. The best clue to his dependence is his refusal to take responsibility for his own care, instead insisting on frequent visits to the doctor, asking the doctor to fill out all the necessary forms, and generally whining and exhorting the doctor to get him well.

This patient also refuses to stop taking drugs. His best hope for successful treatment is the combination of therapies that is offered at a multidisciplinary pain-treatment center (see Chapter 7); more than one admission to such a center may be necessary. The treatment goal for this type of patient is withdrawal from drugs and an increase in activity.

Carol is a middle-aged woman, married for twenty years to a truck driver. Until her accident three years ago, she had worked as a checker in a grocery store. One day on her way to work she hurt herself when she tripped and fell. When she arrived at the store she was covered with bruises from her neck to her lower back. At the urging of her supervisor, she went over to the local hospital where it was discovered that she had ruptured a disc. The disc was repaired in an operation, and Carol said later that the pain cleared up in her mid-back. Yet she complained that the pain in her lower back, shoulder, and neck continued to bother her.

Before her injuries Carol had had a good sexual relationship with her husband, even though he was often away from home on business. She was brought up in a strict Catholic home and got married four years after high school. Her husband was the only man she had ever dated.

After her injury she not only was unable to work but her sex activity had diminished—because, she said, the pain made sex difficult and uncomfortable, and sex made the pain worse.

Carol asked her sister to help out in her home—the pain also prevented her from cooking and doing the housework. She gained thirty-five pounds after her injury and confided to her sister that if it weren't for Valium and Percodan, she couldn't make it through a day.

Carol's doctor referred her to a pain-treatment center where, though she was a congenial personality on the ward, she refused to participate in the recommended exercise program, and she was resistant to being withdrawn from her drugs. During the group therapy sessions she said that the pain did not depress her, but she admitted that she was upset with her husband and wished that he would take care of her as she had taken care of him all those years he was on the road and coming home only briefly and occasionally. She was angry with him, she told the group, but she was unable to tell him about her anger.

The physicians at the treatment center recommended that she have a denervation, which helped her low-back and neck pain. She eventually was withdrawn from drugs and was sent home, still complaining.

Six months later she was back at the treatment center complaining even more bitterly of low-back pain. Her "friends" Valium and Percodan once more were a part of her daily diet.

During a group session this time she admitted that she was afraid that her husband was leaving her and that all his traveling was a means of getting away from her without divorcing her. She also participated more willingly in the recommended therapy on this second go round. She exercised as she was told and began to withdraw from drugs. She received another denervation, this time in her lumbar region (lower back) and this gave her "50 percent" relief. She said that she could live with that.

When she went home, she encouraged and succeeded in getting her husband to join her in family therapy and in nine months she was free from drugs, had lost twenty pounds, and her husband had given up cross-country trucking for a local job, which was a considerable help to her therapy.

The group of exaggerators includes a personality we'll call the histrionic. According to recent research, *** nearly 95% of this personality type are female and they display overdramatic, over-theatrical speech and behavior.

The histrionic person does not form long-term relationships and may, in fact, have a string of divorces or one-night stands as part of her medical history. This person exaggerates her pain verbally rather than in how she perceives it. She uses wild and excessive adjectives. If hospitalized, she rarely looks ill; rather she looks as though she just stepped out of a hairdresser's salon; she also wears revealing or sexy clothing.

This type of pain-patient personality has a need to be the center of attention and uses her looks and an overdramatization of her circumstances to fulfill this need. Her pain is a perfect device for manipulating family, friends, and physician.

When trying to diagnose this type of patient, the doctor will discover some evidence of an organic source for the pain, yet he will not find any signs of depression or anxiety on psychological tests.

This exaggerator needs any and all treatment that the pain-treatment center can offer. Efforts must be made to alter the patient's response to chronic pain, using behavior modification, group therapy, and low doses of mood-affecting drugs. Surgical procedures, other than denervation, probably will not help her because of her personality quirks. Surgery might just give rise to

*** cf. Kaminsky, M. J., and Slavney, P. R., "Methodology and Personality in Briquet's Syndrome, a Reappraisal," *American Journal of Psychiatry,* 1976.

more drama and more expression of pain. By keeping the patient a patient, he remains the center of attention.

Linda is an example of a histrionic personality whose pain turns her into an exaggerator-type chronic-pain patient. She is a thirtyish housewife, married three times, who complains of pain in her shoulders that radiates down to her chest. The pain gradually developed over the last three years, and she says it is worse when she moves things or lifts her arms. Both a neurosurgeon and an orthopedic surgeon examined her and were not able to find anything wrong.

When the pain first started, her family physician prescribed Valium, and then Percodan when it failed to "ease up." After he had tried everything he knew of to find the cause of the pain, he suggested that she see a psychiatrist.

When Linda talked with the psychiatrist, she told him that she was beginning to hate all doctors. They didn't seem to understand that the pain was unbearable and excruciating to the point of being disastrous to her life. However, she also remarked that she had no trouble falling asleep, that she was not depressed, and that the pain had not affected her incredibly wonderful sex life at all.

During her therapy session with the psychiatrist, he noted that she always dressed as if she were going to a formal dance, wearing excessive evening makeup and low-cut blouses or revealing shirts. She always complimented the doctor on his abilities, saying that she was certain that he would help her get rid of the pain.

She also told the therapist that her husband, a successful businessman who traveled a lot, bought her every luxury imaginable and even took her with him to other cities so that she could see doctors there about her pain. She admitted that when her husband was home, she would ask him to rub her neck and this action seemed to ease the pain. At one session that her husband attended, he told the therapist that he felt sorry for Linda because she always seemed to be in so much pain, and that he now stayed home more often in order to be with her.

Linda entered a pain treatment center. She refused to give up Percodan although she agreed to switch from Valium to a mood elevator. She also tried a transcutaneous stimulator (see Chapter 6). But after two months she continued to complain that she was in pain, that the new medications were not helping her, and the stimulator was more of an irritant than a soother. She was released, but several months later she came back to the treatment center, where once again she refused to be withdrawn from Percodan; the staff even suspected that somehow she was hoarding other narcotics smuggled in by friends. Again she left the center but continued with group therapy once a week.

After several months, Linda began to comply with some of the suggestions that the group and her psychiatrist made, and she participated in physical therapy. She began to go out more with her husband, even though the pain, she said, hurt like the devil.

With the help of her therapy, she eventually changed her attitude and now uses her story of triumph over the pain as a way of impressing all her friends, or manipulating them, and thus eliciting their approval of her new behavior—being pain free.

There is another Type II personality who does not exactly exaggerate his pain. This person is absorbed in his pain, is fascinated by it, much as someone is fascinated or absorbed by a glowing fire. This person is a victim of what psychiatrists call Briquet's syndrome.

Before the onset of pain, this Type II personality has already shown that he does not adjust well to life's stresses. He has a long history of not feeling well, of having headaches and fatigue, anxiety, sexual difficulties, and bowel problems.

The patient is usually a woman who has had many divorces or broken engagements. Chronic pain takes her by surprise. It usually is general and vague and difficult to describe in words to the doctor.

The onset pain often sends her to bed—where, if possible, she remains. The pain does not interfere with her sleep, but her sex activity is diminished. She starts abusing any pill she can lay her hands on, including laxatives.

Physicians can diagnose Briquet's syndrome by using a checklist. In most cases the patient can identify at least twenty-five symptoms that she is suffering from in a list of fifty-five, yet the symptoms have never been diagnosed. By the age of thirty-five, she will also have a long and complicated medical history that matches the list of symptoms.

Some of the symptoms that the Briquet's syndrome patient will claim to suffer from (besides vague pain) include: feeling sickly most of her life, headaches, blindness, unconsciousness, fits, convulsions, amnesia, deafness, hallucinations, fatigue, lump in the throat, fainting spells, visual blurring, weakness, thirstiness, palpitations, chest pain, dizziness, appetite loss, weight loss, nausea, diarrhea, constipation, menstrual cramps, menstrual irregularities, frigidity, back pain, joint pain, nervousness, and general depressed feelings. (The physician should ascertain whether or not the patient consulted a doctor for the symptoms she claims so that he can make a determination as to whether the symptoms should count toward diagnosis.)

Because this patient is plagued with a variety of symptoms and frequently complains about the intensity of the pain associated with each one, her treatment is usually not directed at her symptoms but at teaching her to deal or cope with reality. This Type II personality should never be challenged about the validity of any of her symptoms or the intensity of her pain (even if it seems that the patient is a malingerer without any pain). Treatment can range from the use of placebos (sugar pills) to family therapy, group therapy, electroconvulsive therapy (shock treatment), or sleep therapy. Hospitalization in a pain-treatment center where a range of these therapies is offered can be beneficial to this type.

Until the treating physician convinces the patient that he believes that the pain is real, however, therapy probably will fail. A Briquet's syndrome patient takes a lack of belief as a challenge—and she probably will not get well.

Paula is a fifty-three-year-old patient with Briquet's syndrome who also suffers from chronic pain in her shoulder and neck and occasional severe headaches. Most of the tests performed on her indicate that she is a healthy woman, although she does show some signs of osteoporosis (a softening of the bones, usually due to old age).

Paula said that the onset of her pain was gradual and that it made it difficult for her to fall asleep and was interfering with her work as an interior decorator. She had had no sex life to speak of before the pain, so it did not affect this area of her life.

Paula's medical record was as thick as a telephone book. She had more than forty hospitalizations, including three face-lifts, reconstructive surgery on her jaw, a gallbladder removal, and hysterectomy all before the age of forty. Her record also listed many emergency room visits for sprains and broken bones sustained during unexplained falls. She was taking almost every over-the-counter medication on the market, including massive doses of multiple vitamins. She also was taking prescription drugs, including thyroid medication, a diuretic, and amphetamines for her multiple crash diets.

When the pain first started bothering her on the job, she visited three doctors, who only glanced at her medical records and told her it was all in her head. Even her son, a physician, said he did not believe that she was in "real" pain.

Paula was finally referred to a therapist who believed her pain was real and that she was suffering. He took her off most of her vitamins and all the prescription drugs and gave her a transcutaneous stimulator (a device to block pain; see Chapter 6).

Within three months she said that the pain was under control. She stopped seeing the psychotherapist at this time and joined a church that advocated a holistic medicine philosophy—combining medicine with religious faith. Because the holistic people all said that they believed in her pain and understood her problems, she said, her pain completely went away.

When psychosomatic disorders contribute to the poor premorbid adjustment of an exaggerator, the first thing the patient will tell the doctor is that he is high-strung. He will also have a history of marital discord, sexual difficulties, financial disasters, tension, anxiety, and nervousness. He will say that the reason for any one of these problems is that he is under a lot of pressure, either at home or at work, and he never has time to relax or enjoy a hobby. He describes his pain as a tightness in the neck or shoulder muscles. He might have facial pain, low-back pain, or a headache over his eyes. His pain developed slowly, no accident or trauma can be pinpointed as having caused it. The pain interferes with falling asleep, and it interferes with sex.

The nervous tension this patient feels generally translates into physical tension, and this translates into pain. Heat and massage may relieve the pain, as will certain neurolytic drugs, which will reduce his anxiety. Supportive psychotherapy is useful for this type of patient, particularly therapy that involves other family members.

Mary is a forty-two-year-old woman who grew up feeling the effects of the Depression. Her parents never failed to remind her how much they had to sacrifice in order to bring her into the world. Her husband, a construction worker, had been laid off for several months every year for the last six years. Mary took a job waitressing, even though her husband objected to her working.

About four years ago Mary started having facial pain under her cheekbones that radiated toward her ear, and even bothered her jaws at times. After waiting four years, she finally thought she could afford to go see a doctor.

She told the physician about the pain and also said she had pain in her neck and shoulders. She admitted that she felt a great deal of tension, at home from arguments with her husband and at work from her customers. She told him she had trouble sleeping at night but the pain did not interfere with her sex life. She had visited a local emergency room several years before and received prescriptions for Darvon and Librium, and these gave her some relief.

The physician, after hearing her symptoms, suggested that she see a dentist, something she hadn't done since her husband began receiving his periodic layoffs. The dentist diagnosed Mary as having temporomandibular joint syndrome. Her physician then made her stop taking the Darvon and Librium and started her on neuroleptic, muscle relaxant, and anti-inflammatory drugs. Within two weeks her pain was diminished.

On her dentist's recommendation, Mary entered the hospital in order to have her bite repositioned; it was so severely out of line that the dentist thought it had contributed to her pain. After a three-week hospital stay, she was virtually pain-free due to the dental surgery as well as Mary's having learned how to reduce her tension by relaxing her bite. Over time, her neck and shoulder pain also diminished—as did her tension.

Type III, the Mopers

The moper is a third category of pain patient who experiences chronic pain in his own peculiar way. This patient is very similar to Type I (the coper) except the cause for his pain is unknown, and this fills him with anxiety and fear—he frets or mopes about what can possibly be wrong with him.

This type of patient is particularly trying to the physician because no cause can be found for his pain, and the patient is not known to be a complainer. The physician is often tempted to refer the moper to a psychiatrist. However, if the physician looks at the patient's premorbid adjustment, he will find him to be a stable personality who seems to have nothing to gain from chronic pain. Nor is the moper known to be a manipulator who might use the pain as a means of getting attention.

Kent is a middle-aged man who is a production supervisor at a paint manufacturing company. He has been married to the same woman for more than thirty years and has two children.

For six years Kent complained of pain on the left side of his chest near his nipple and under his rib. His family doctor ran tests for pancreatitis, arthritis, and neuralgia, and they all came back negative. He was given a local anesthesia (anesthesia injected into the skin), and all that happened was that his skin turned numb at the injection site. He received no relief from the pain. Every day that the pain bothered him, it bothered him in the same place, and he never changed his story except to say that the pain varied in intensity.

Kent eventually was referred to a psychiatrist who noted that he had had a good pre-pain adjustment, that his marriage was solid, that he had a good job he claimed he liked, that his children were well-adjusted, and that he had a few interests outside of work, such as hunting. Kent told the psychiatrist that he did have trouble falling asleep (he often wondered whether he had cancer and no one was telling him) and that sometimes he was awakened by pain—on the average of three or four times a week for the last three years.

Throughout his years of pain, Kent managed to remain free from drug addiction—though it was hard, he admitted. He tried to kill the pain with aspirin, but this medication did not help very much, and lately the constant ache had been making him very depressed. Because he was depressed, he was not working very well, and at home, he found that he did not have much interest in sex anymore. In general, life did not seem pleasant. He even found that hunting, his favorite sport, no longer held any interest for him because he couldn't concentrate on what he was doing.

During a visit to a neurosurgeon, an office nurse said that she thought she felt a swollen nodule on his rib on the side of his chest, but the neurosurgeon detected nothing, nor did an orthopedic surgeon who was called in as a consultant. Kent's psychiatrist, however, with the aid of thermography, detected an area of pain in the place Kent said ached constantly. The area was then injected with steroids and the pain disappeared in two days.

Within three months Kent said that he no longer felt depressed, and he felt his interest ignite once again in sex, hunting, and work.

Type IV, the Malingerers (conscious and unconscious)

This last group of patients includes people who truly have no pain. They use the memory of some previous pain to describe their current ("imaginary") pain.

Some of the Type IV patients out-and-out lie about what they are feeling. They say they are in pain, knowing full well they are not. They are conscious malingerers. Others may say they are in pain when they are not, but they are not really lying—they are more likely having a problem in perception. These are people with either severe emotional trauma associated with the injury, or a psychiatric disease that alters their perception of reality. One might call these unconscious malingerers.

Conscious malingerers find pain to be useful; they say they have it in order to use it. Unconscious malingerers have some psychological reason for their pain; there is no malicious intent behind the complaints. Whether or not the malingerer is aware of his reason for saying he is in pain when he is not is an essential distinction physicians need to make before prescribing treatment.

The person who unconsciously uses his "pain" has "converted" the problem into "pain." Conversion is an unconscious defense mechanism that some people use to protect themselves from life's stresses, particularly the stresses that they perceive as overwhelming or unacceptable. However, pain is rarely, if ever, used as a "conversion" symptom, since it is not visible to others. You can't get attention from something that is invisible.

There is also another type of patient who fits into this fourth category: the person who suffers from delusional thinking. The pain in this case is incorrectly perceived. This misperception is neither conscious nor unconscious; it is a manifestation of an inability to correctly sort through one's thoughts and feelings. True malingering, on the other hand, is a *conscious* effort to deceive someone, whether family members, an organization or business, or insurance company.

Surgeons in particular should beware of Type IV patients; they may convince the doctor that surgery is important and desirable when it is actually the worst thing that could be done for or to them. They are a difficult group of people to identify, especially delusionals, because delusions are real to the person who is affected with a thinking disorder. (Sometimes an exaggerator may be targeted as a malingerer. The difference between the two, however, is that there is usually an organic lesion or obscure disease affecting the exaggerator, which thorough testing should eventually identify.)

How do you determine whether a person is malingering? Once again, you look at the premorbid adjustment.

The malingerer is a person who has tried to deceive other people all his life. He may have an arrest record or a history of drug addiction. If he is in constant financial trouble, he may see malingering as a way to help him out of his problems by qualifying him to collect unemployment insurance, Social Security disability payments, or workmen's compensation. Yet, it is hard to pick out a malingerer from past history alone, as he is more prone to fake an illness when his circumstances call for it, when he sees sickness or pain as a way out of a sticky situation. He may view his deception as self-preservation rather than a dishonest way of getting attention or easy money.

There are some family and environmental situations that may help propel someone along the path to malingering. A person who comes from a poor family, especially a poor and large family, may resort to malingering in order to escape responsibilities or duties that he does not like.

A malingerer usually makes a great show of his "disability," but it is difficult to remember to keep limping or not use a particular arm. Pain, however, is the ideal symptom, as there is no way to measure pain, and a physician can only proceed on the basis that the patient says he is in pain. If the patient is examined closely, however, the physician will see that there is no muscle atrophy (wasting away from disuse), although the patient claims he never uses that limb or part of his body anymore. The malingerer doesn't get better over any period of time, nor does his "disease" get worse in any way.

Though difficult to diagnose, there are ways that a malingerer can be discovered. After a meticulous examination, during which the doctor or examiner maintains an unbiased nonjudgmental attitude, the doctor should initiate a discussion with the patient, allowing him to talk about his fears, his problems, and anything that concerns him about his treatment.

The physician also should try to find out whether or not the patient consulted his attorney before he came for medical treatment. He should compare the symptoms the patient presents at one session to those he presents at the next and ascertain whether there are any gross contradictions.

The malingerer may avoid answering questions or submitting to examinations. In this case the examiner should note whether or not the patient is able to pursue his hobbies, although he no longer works or maintains his household responsibilities. By putting all these observations together, the true malingerer may be detected.

Treatment of this type of patient is difficult. Surgery is obviously not going to be helpful, and therapy most likely will be useless, although family therapy might be helpful. Benign neglect, without confronting the patient with his fakery, is a possible course of action.

Surprisingly, a cash settlement may not even cure the malingerer, especially if he has found his pain or condition useful on the home front.

Ron is a thirty-five-year-old janitor who is married and has four children. He is not particularly fond of his job working in a factory; most days he is bored with it and resentful that he has to work the early shift. He has always hated getting up at or before dawn.

One day soon after he arrived at work and punched in, he lifted a heavy box to toss into the trash bin and suddenly felt a pain in his lower back. He immediately went to his supervisor and told him that he thought he had strained his back while lifting the trash.

Ron's supervisor sent him to the company doctor, who told Ron to take the rest of the day off and spend a couple of days in bed, just resting. While he was at home, Ron called his cousin, an attorney, because his union steward told him that the company ought to do something for him other than sending him home for a few days. After talking with his cousin, Ron started to put together some information that he could use in order to get workmen's compensation.

Ron told the Workmen's Compensation Board that the pain in his back was so bad that he could not work and he could not have sex with his wife anymore. The board granted him compensation, as did Social Security (which he also contacted within a day of his injury). Ron now had more income than he ever had from his job as a janitor.

Since he was not working at the factory, but had all that money coming in, Ron decided to use his leisure time constructively and take a course in appliance repair. Meanwhile, he had to return to the company doctor for a periodic physical examination under orders of the Workmen's Compensation Board. The doctor listened to Ron's complaints of pain and noted that he was able to lift his legs while seated but not when he was lying down. The doctor sent him to another board physician for a psychiatric evaluation, which showed him to be a passive person with some anxieties and depression. The board decided that Ron should return to work.

At the same time, the factory's insurance company was working hard to determine whether or not his claim should be paid, and it hired an investigator to spy on Ron. Using hidden cameras, the insurance people found that he could lift heavy boxes when no one was around and that he also rode a motorcycle when he thought no one he knew was watching. Ron did not seem to be in any pain when he was lifting those boxes or riding the motorcycle. He was asked to see the psychiatrist once more.

Because the doctor seemed to be sympathetic, Ron tearfully admitted that it was not so much that he was in pain but that he could never handle the work load that was assigned to him, and he was afraid his fellow workers would laugh at him and think he was a sissy if they knew that. Ron also admitted that he didn't have sex with his wife anymore because she had gained about fifty pounds after her last pregnancy and had never taken it off. Fat people always repulsed him, he said.

After counseling, Ron agreed to undergo psychotherapy with his wife and participate in vocational rehabilitation. After job retraining, and after his wife had lost forty pounds, Ron quit collecting disability payments and went to work again—in an appliance store.

Ron was a case of malingering. He used his pain to get out of a stressful situation at work and used it to leave the workplace that he did not like. He found that it was also useful at home as a weapon against his wife's "repulsive" fat. Once the home and work situations were resolved to his satisfaction, his pain also was resolved.

The Type IV personality whose pain is due to conversion or delusion is not as easy a case to help. There are so few cases of personalities like his that it is difficult for doctors to properly diagnose his symptoms.

Conversion is a difficult process to understand and can easily mask many other psychiatric or organic ailments. Even people who are considered "normal" in every way may experience conversion symptoms during overwhelmingly stressful times—especially after a traumatic incident. For example, the wife who is driving the car when there is an accident that kills her passenger—her husband—may convert her grief and guilt into an excruciating back or neck pain.

There is no typical premorbid adjustment for the personality that converts life stresses or traumas into pain. This is because conversion is usually an unexpected consequence—it represents a method of coping. Because it is an unconscious event, the person believes and is convinced that the pain is real. This is not to say that the pain is imaginary—there is no imaginary pain. What happens with the patient who experiences conversion is that he perceives pain, but pain that is strictly related to an emotional event and not to any organic source. The pain is real in that it probably hurts, but it is only real as long as the patient needs it as a coping mechanism. Treatment for this kind of pain includes the use of psychotherapy and mood-elevating drugs. Sometimes electroconvulsive therapy is prescribed.

Frieda is a fortyish computer programmer, a fuss budget who demands perfection from herself in all phases of her life. She was divorced abruptly after a ten-year marriage because she felt that she and her husband were incompatible.

About one month after an auto accident Frieda started complaining about a headache at the back of her head. She also claimed that she was losing her ability to concentrate and to calculate figures, a necessary part of her job.

When she went to see a doctor for the headaches, he took a brain-wave test (EEG) and several other neurological tests and found them all to be normal. While taking her history, the doctor learned that she had suffered a depression after her divorce and that she had gone into therapy briefly for it.

Frieda admitted to her physician that she was compulsive about her job, but she also said that the job required a great deal of fastidiousness. She told him she was depressed most of the time now that she had the pain, and she had trouble falling asleep.

The doctor believed that these problems might be the result of a concussion Frieda had suffered in the accident and prescribed some mood elevators for her. But Frieda still did not feel well, and she quit work because she claimed that her difficulty in concentration did not allow her to run programs properly.

After three months of drug therapy Frieda said that her concentration was improved and she was working part time. Since she was afraid of making mistakes, she did not feel ready to return to work full time.

During her part-time employment, she was trying to sue the person who had hit her car. She found out that he was uninsured and had left the state because the police were going to arrest him for other misdemeanors on his record (he was out on bail at the time of the car accident). Frieda told her doctor that she knew that she would never collect from him, and she felt that he and the insurance company cheated her. Frieda decided to enter into psychotherapy on the suggestion of her doctor.

Though she admitted during therapy sessions that she was afraid of dying in an auto accident, and was terribly shaken by her recent one, the catharsis of her admission did not help her to get rid of her headaches. However, during one of her sessions, after a year in therapy, Frieda recalled an incident from an experience in her childhood: her mother had hit her on the back of her head because she had refused to tie her shoes. She immediately realized that the blow she had received from her mother felt exactly like the blow she had suffered during the car accident. And when she was a child, she remembered, she had been frustrated that she was unable to hit back at her mother for what she considered to be an unjust punishment. She felt the same way about the driver who had hit her and fled the state without paying for the damages on her car. Just as she had wanted to kill her mother for the blow on the head, she also wanted to kill the driver for destroying her car and, in part, her life (her ability to concentrate). In front of her therapist, she burst into tears. The following week her headaches virtually disappeared.

Chronic pain is difficult to diagnose and difficult to treat. It is as diverse as the personalities of the people who complain of it.

No matter what the cause of the pain (although it usually has an organic basis), the personality of the patient has an overwhelming effect on his treatment and on how quickly or slowly he progresses. If he really wants to get better and return to his life as it was before the pain, he has a good chance of succeeding. If he has found a special use for his pain, the most sophisticated drugs and devices may not alleviate it.

All pain (except in the case of the conscious malingerer) is perceived as real to the person who is suffering it. This must be accepted by all involved in the pain treatment—the physician as well as the patient.

Coping with chronic pain may be easier for you knowing that there are others like you. The realization that even the coper has a difficult time adjusting to it and living with it may be comforting. A close examination of your own personality may help you to ascertain its effects on the role pain plays in your life.

5
Diagnosing Pain

Diagnosing the underlying cause of chronic pain is at best difficult. Since pain is a subjective experience, the use of objective, quantifying tests (such as asking *how much* does it hurt) is inadequate.

Standard diagnostic tools such as X-rays, electromyographic studies (tests of muscle power or strength), nerve-conduction studies (how well the nerve performs its duties), and physical exams can pinpoint organic causes of pain complaints. These tests can find lesions on nerves, degenerating muscles, inflammation of joints, the imbalances of fluids in the body—all of which cause pain. The many pain syndromes, however, are obscure and not well publicized in the medical literature. These syndromes include myofascial pain, temporomandibular-joint syndrome, and sympathetic dystrophies. The old standby tests such as the physical exam, nerve-conduction studies, etc., are good as far as they go, but they don't take into account the special problems of a patient suffering from pain the source of which is hard to isolate and they don't take into account the fact that chronic pain is a disease in itself.

A simple psychological screening exam is one way of clarifying some chronic-pain problems. Often patients afflicted with the more obscure organically caused pain syndromes have spent a lot of time on a psychiatrist's couch or in sessions with a psychologist because they have been told their pain is only imaginary, that it is all in their heads.

You may have already encountered some tests that are used to analyze a variety of complaints from people, including chronic-pain patients, who seek psychiatric help. One of the most common screening tests for personality disorders or for simple personality evaluation is the Minnesota Multiphasic Personality Inventory (MMPI), which contains nearly six-hundred true or false questions that a person answers himself. Another screening test that is coming into vogue is the SCL 90-R, a ninety-question test which again is answered on a score sheet.

Based on the results of the MMPI, psychiatrists and psychologists determine the personality traits of their patients. In particular, the MMPI picks out such characteristics as hysteria or tendency to hypochondria, or it determines whether or not the patient is anxious or depressed. Some scientists and physicians use this test to predict the outcome of treatment: how well a person will respond to treatment, if he will recover (particularly pertinent in the case of a preoperative patient).

Some physicians believe, however, that the MMPI is an invalid tool for diagnosing chronic-pain patients because although it has built-in safeguards against internal inconsistencies the test does not take into account personality factors that change over time. Filling in an answer sheet without supervision allows the patient to interpret the questions as he wishes, and this leaves room for misinterpretation of the intent of the questions. The patient may also prejudge his answer before he puts it down and decide that another response might show him in a better light, thereby skewing his score. Also, the test is not specifically designed for pain patients.

The SCL 90-R, created by Leonard Derogatis, Ph.D., at Johns Hopkins Hospital, evaluates complaints over a period of time. The test is a list of problems and complaints, ranging from headaches, faintness, or dizziness, to the feeling that people are unfriendly and don't like you. The patient marks the ninety statements to indicate how much discomfort ("not at all," "a little bit," "a great deal") any particular problem has caused him over a period of time, up to and including the day of the test. This test has its limitations too, since it requires the patient to judge how he feels, subject to his own interpretation, rather than the observations of a trained clinician. However, it has the advantage of being able to assess changes in a person's feelings over time.

Some pain-treatment clinics develop their own diagnostic tests based on past experience with their patients. These tests usually incorporate the best features of those mentioned above and include innovative questions devised by the staff based on their observations of former pain patients. One such example is a ten-minute-screening test for chronic back-pain patients developed at the Johns Hopkins Chronic Pain Treatment Center by Dr. Nelson Hendler in conjunction with Dr. Donlin Long, the center's director and professor of neurosurgery at the hospital.

Thermography, one of the "new" diagnostic *devices,* actually has been around for some time, but it has been used in the past to diagnose breast cancer and other abnormalities of the breast. Thermography detects breast disease by measuring the heat that the breast tissue gives off. If there is abnormal tissue in the breast, such as cysts or tumors, the thermograph will confirm this by registering higher temperatures in these areas than in the rest of the breast.

This process varies for pain patients, depending on the disorder. If there is reduced blood flow causing the pain, thermography will register the painful area as a cool spot. In one East Coast pain clinic, thermography has revealed the presence of pain in nearly one third of the cases when previous tests indicated that the problem had no organic source. One patient who had severe facial pain looked at his thermograph showing areas of both heat and cold and said that it was a map of his pain.

Thermography has been most helpful when the pain is caused by a change in or trauma to the sympathetic nerves. The thermograph can direct the physician to the appropriate ganglions (nerve bundles) or chain of nerves that need blocking or denervation.

When a patient checks into a clinic that provides thermographic diagnosis, he will be taken to a special room where his body can adjust to the room air temperature. The portion of his body affected by the pain—lower or upper—will be exposed to the air. After about fifteen minutes of exposure the thermographic unit will be trained on his body; at the same time the thermograph is in operation, a Polaroid picture is taken. It is this picture that delineates the "map" of his pain.

In the picture, light areas correspond to warm regions and dark areas to cool regions of the body. Differences in temperature are measured by comparing anatomically identical areas of opposite parts of the body: if, for example, the pain is in your right arm, pictures of both that arm and the left arm are taken; these two pictures showing light and dark areas are then compared.

Scientists speculate that areas of pain show up as cool spots because of vasoconstriction, the squeezing shut of blood vessels. This stricture shuts off the supply of blood to the area, cutting off the oxygen supply that is carried by the blood and thereby lowering the temperature of the area that is the source of the pain.

Another device, barely three years in general use, is the computed tomographic scanner, better known as the CAT scanner, but more accurately referred to as a CT scanner.

The CT scanner is an X-ray device (it looks like a futuristic coffin made of steel and attached to rotating platforms) that uses computers, X-rays, and Polaroid-type pictures to give cross-section views of all parts of the body, including the brain. Viewing these cross sections is like looking at the individual slices of a loaf of bread. In other words, physicians can see various cross-sections of an organ, not just the outline or silhouette. The CT whole-body scanner and the CT brain scanner can detect lesions that are difficult for X-rays to define. The scan is particularly useful for brain conditions and detecting problems in the abdominal cavity.

A thorough diagnosis, which includes diagnosis of personality type and how it affects the chronic-pain patient's outlook on life, is the prelude to treatment.

How Much Pain Do You Feel? A Test for Pain Victims

The following Screening Test for Chronic Back Pain Patients is designed to screen patients for the purpose of facilitating appropriate treatment decisions. As a pain victim, you also will be able to see how you handle chronic pain and how pain affects you. The test should take you about ten minutes to complete. For each question circle the statement that most closely applies to you, and mark down the number of points you receive on a separate sheet of paper. This test is specifically designed for back pain and may not accurately reflect responses to other types of pain.

I When did you first notice the pain that you now experience?
- (a) Sudden onset after/with an accident or definable event. 0
- (b) Slow, progressive onset, with sharp accompanying pain. 1
- (c) Slow, progressive onset, without sharp accompanying pain. 2
- d) A sudden onset of pain without an accident or event to which you can tie the pain. 3

II Where do you feel the pain?
- (a) One specific, well-defined place. 0
- (b) Several different places. 1
- (c) One place, but hard to tell exactly where. 2
- (d) It's hard to describe exactly where the pain is, and it feels different in different places. No physician has been able to tie it to a specific source. 3

III Do you have trouble falling asleep at night?
No. (If no, go to question V.) 3
Yes. (If yes, go to question IV.) 4

IV What keeps you from falling asleep at night?
- (a) I have trouble falling asleep at night because of pain, and I'm awakened by the pain every night. 0

(b) Because of the pain, I have trouble falling asleep about three times a week or more, and I'm awakened by the pain from sleep more than three times a week. 1
(c) I have trouble falling asleep more than three times a week, but I'm not awakened from sleep by the pain more than twice a week. 2
(d) I have no trouble falling asleep because of the pain, and it does not wake me once I'm asleep. 3
(e) I have trouble falling asleep, or I'm awakened early in the morning—but it's not because of the pain. 4

V Does the weather have any effect on your pain?
(a) The pain is always worse with *both* cold and damp weather. 0
(b) The pain is always worse with *either* damp or cold weather. 1
(c) The pain is occasionally worse with cold or damp weather. 2
(d) The weather has no effect on the pain. 3

VI How would you describe the type of pain you have now?
(a) Burning, or sharp, shooting pain, or pins and needles, or coldness, or numbness. 0
(b) Dull, aching pain, with occasional sharp shooting pains, not helped by heat applications; or abnormal sense of cold or heat to touch. 1
(c) Spasm-type pain, tension-type pain, or a numbness over the area of pain helped by massage and heat. 2
(d) Nagging or bothersome pain. 3
(e) Excruciating, overwhelming, or unbearable pain, relieved by heat or massage. 4

VII How frequently do you have pain?
(a) The pain is constant. 0
(b) The pain is nearly constant, 50%–80% of the time. 1
(c) The pain is intermittent, 25%–50% of the time. 2
(d) The pain is only occasionally present, less than 25% of the time. 3

VIII Does movement or position have any effect on the pain?

(a) The pain is unrelieved by a position change or when I don't use that part of my body where it hurts. I also have a history of previous operations for the pain. 0

(b) The pain gets worse when I use that part of my body where it hurts or when I stand or walk. It's relieved when I lie down, or when I don't use that part of my body where it hurts. 1

(c) The pain is affected according to my position or my use of the part of my body where it hurts. 2

(d) There is no change in the pain with a change in position or use of the part of my body where it hurts. I have not had any operations for the pain. 3

IX What medications have you used in the past month?

(a) No medication at all. 0

(b) I've used a non-narcotic pain reliever or a mild tranquilizer (non-benzodiazepam) or an antidepressant. 1

(c) I've used a strong pain-killer or a sleeping pill less than three times a week, or I've taken a (benzodiazepam) tranquilizer less than three times a week. 2

(d) I've used either a pain-killer or a sleeping pill or a tranquilizer (benzodiazepam) more than four times a week. 3

X What hobbies do you have? Can you still participate in them?

(a) I am unable to participate at all in any hobbies I used to enjoy. 0

(b) I've reduced my number of hobbies or activities relating to the hobbies. 1

(c) I still participate in my hobbies, but with some discomfort. 2

(d) I participate in my hobbies the same as before. 3

XI How frequently did you have sex and orgasms before the pain? How frequently do you have sex and orgasms now?

(a) I had a good sexual relationship prior to the pain,

about three or four times a week, with no difficulty with orgasm, but now I have sexual contacts less than once a week and that is interrupted by pain. 0

(b) Before the pain, I had a good sexual relationship, about three or four times a week, with no difficulty with orgasms, but now I have less interest in sex, have sex less than once a week, and have difficulty with orgasm or erection. 1

(c) There has been no change in my sexual activity. It is the same now as it was before I began experiencing the pain. 2

(d) I am unable to have any sexual contact since the pain, and I had difficulty with orgasms or erection prior to the pain. 3

XII Are you still working or doing your household chores?

(a) I work every day at the same job I had prior to the onset of my pain, at the same level and with the same duties. 0

(b) I work every day, but the job is not the same as I had before the onset of pain. I have reduced responsibilities or fewer activities. 1

(c) I work sporadically, or I have reduced my household chores. 2

(d) I don't work any more, or someone else does my household chores. 3

XIII What is your income now compared to the time before your injury or the beginning of your pain? What are the sources of your income?

(a) I'm experiencing financial difficulty, and my family income has been cut in half or more since the onset of the pain. 0

(b) I'm experiencing some financial difficulty, with my family income 50%–75% of the pre-pain income. 1

(c) I am unable to work; I receive some compensation and my spouse works, so my income is at least 75% of my pre-pain income. 2

(d) My income is about 80% or more than my gross pay before the pain, and my spouse does not work. 3

XIV Are you suing anyone, or is anyone suing you, or do you

have an attorney helping you with compensation or disability payment?

(a) I have no suits pending, and I do not have an attorney. 0

(b) I have a suit pending, but it is not related to the pain. 1

(c) I am being sued as the result of an accident. 2

(d) I have a suit pending, or I am expecting workmen's compensation, and I have a lawyer involved. 3

XV If you had three wishes for anything in the world, what would you wish for?

(a) "Get rid of the pain" is the only wish I would have for all three wishes. 0

(b) "Get rid of the pain" would be one of my three wishes. 1

(c) My wishes would be something of a personal nature, such as having more money, having a better relationship with my spouse or my children, and having a bigger house. 2

(d) My wishes would be for something like peace in the world, an end to hunger, or something else for others. 3

XVI Have you ever been depressed or thought of suicide?

(a) I have been depressed, or I have been depressed in addition to having pain. My depression makes me cry at times or think of suicide. 0

(b) Because of the pain, I've been depressed, and I've felt guilty and angry. 1

(c) I felt depressed before the pain, or before the pain I suffered a financial or personal loss (death of a friend, family member moved away), and now with the pain here, I also have some depression. 2

(d) I don't feel depressed, I don't have crying jags, or I don't feel blue. 3

(e) Before the pain I had a history of suicide attempts. 4

Add up all your points. A score of 18 points or less suggests that you are a Type I personality (a coper) and are showing the normal response to chronic pain. You are usually willing to participate in suggested therapy, including exercise and supportive psychotherapy.

A score of 19–31 points suggests that you are a Type II personality (the exaggerator). Surgical or other intervention procedures may be recommended for you with caution. The test shows that you may have found a use for chronic pain. You may benefit from treatment at a chronic-pain center with an emphasis on attitude change toward the chronic pain.

A score of 32 points or more suggests that a psychiatric consultation is needed. You are the type of personality that freely admits that you had a great many pre-pain problems and that you have a great deal of difficulty coping with the chronic pain you now have. Surgical or other intervention procedures should not be carried out without prior approval of a psychiatric consultant.

6
Therapies and Treatments to Help You Cope

Pain therapy can involve any of the following treatments, singly or in combination, for any amount of time, from two weeks to several months, to many years: drug withdrawal, the prescription of drugs, surgery, nerve blocks, transcutaneous stimulators, electrical implants, psychotherapy, group therapy, family therapy, occupational therapy, behavior modification, biofeedback, hypnosis, and acupuncture.

Some pain clinics limit themselves to specific kinds of pain or a particular form of therapy: there are clinics that devote themselves exclusively to the treatment of headaches or backaches; there are some clinics that use only anesthetics and others that use only nerve blocks in their therapy. We will talk about the multidisciplinary pain clinic as a mode of pain treatment, as it seems to have the best record in relief proffered and obtained.

A number of these treatments may be available at the private offices of some physical therapists or physicians and at some general hospitals. However, they can be found in the greatest concentration at pain clinics.

Listed below are some of the most widely available treatments in this country today:

Drug Withdrawal

Pain-clinic physicians often request that new patients bring in all the presciption and over-the-counter drugs they are taking at the time of their admission or have taken in the past for their pain. Some patients literally bring in a shopping bag filled with pills and admit to taking all of them. Some of the medications may be harmless. Some may be placebos, sugar pills prescribed by a physician who didn't believe "the pain was real" but wanted to give his patient something to assuage his fears.

Some pills are harmful; they can be addicting, depressing, or even worsen the pain. Some pills, for example, when taken in combination with others, can potentiate the intended effect of both drugs. Potentiation can cause mood changes, body-chemistry changes, coma or death from overdose.

Unfortunately, the most widely prescribed drugs for chronic pain are addicting. Addiction occurs when your body reaches a tolerance level for a prescribed dosage of a drug and then requires a larger dose for it to have the same effect it once had. As you increase your tolerance level, you must ingest more and more of the drug until at last you can't function during the day without it—your body chemistry has been altered and needs it.

If you are addicted to pain-killers, sleeping pills, or tranquilizers, they have probably become part of your daily routine, and you swallow them without thinking. But they might also be contributing to your pain either through a direct effect on your body (where the drugs themselves are causing pain or discomfort) or an incidental side effect (such as when the drugs induce drowsiness keeping you in bed all day when what your body actually needs is physical exercise to help rid itself of the pain). Unfortunately, some of the most widely prescribed drugs, the benzodiazepines (such as Valium and Librium) can be addicting. They are prescribed by well-intentioned doctors to their patients who complain of chronic pain, but in fact may worsen pain.

A vicious circle begins with the first prescription. Benzodiazepines may alleviate anxiety for a time, but never to the root of pain. So when the pain returns, the patient takes more pills, until he or she reaches the point where he takes the pills before the pain comes, because his body requires them.

Barbiturate sleeping pills (such as Seconal or Tuinal) also are frequently prescribed and are easily abused and are addictive. Sleeping pills are prescribed when the patient complains that either he can't get to sleep at night because of the pain or that he has trouble staying asleep. Again the doctor is well-intentioned, but by prescribing sleeping pills he is contributing to the pain-pill cycle. Frequently patients who are "on" sleeping pills need amphetamines to wake them up in the morning, and then they need the sleeping pills at night to counter the effects of the stimulants.

By the time a chronic-pain patient has accumulated a shopping bag filled with pills, his life is built around his medication. When he arrives at the pain clinic, the staff will assess his drugs. They need to see how the patient functions and feels without the pills, so withdrawal is initiated. They need to see his reaction to the pain without the dulling effect of drugs.

For some people withdrawal from drugs may be quite simple. The staff takes away the pills and does not provide any more unless a staff physician orders them. Period. The patient is withdrawn.

For others drug withdrawal may be a slow, gradual process. The body must get accustomed once again to functioning without the pills. Usually the body cannot stand the shock of instant withdrawal (cold turkey). So the treatment center doles the drugs out in increasingly smaller doses until the body can handle not having any drugs at all.

Drug withdrawal is not offered as a sole treatment in a pain clinic. It is an adjunctive therapy. It works best when undertaken voluntarily and with a total commitment.

Prescribing Drugs

Although pain clinics usually advocate withdrawal from all drugs, treatment may consist of a drug regimen. How drugs work and why they are used will be discussed thoroughly in Chapter 9.

Surgery

Surgery is the most complex and serious treatment recommended by pain clinics. Surgery should be avoided if there is some equally effective method of treatment. However, in some cases it is the only means available to conquer chronic pain.

People with trigeminal neuralgia, for example, are often treated with drugs that temporarily control the excruciating pain.

Anticonvulsive drugs such as Dilantin or Tegretol control the agony for a time, but surgery may be called for eventually.

One of the newest procedures developed to aid the victims of the dread tic douloureux is percutaneous rhizotomy (an operation that is, in part, performed on an awake and alert patient). The surgeon guides a needle-thin electrode through the patient's cheek to the appropriate offending nerve. During this procedure the patient is awake so he can tell the surgeon whether he has found the correct nerve. The surgeon then thermocoagulates the nerve (heats the nerve until the pain fibers are destroyed), effectively cutting off the energy supply to the cheek. The thermocoagulation portion of the surgery is performed with the patient under general anesthesia.

As with any operation there are drawbacks because of the potential side effects of the procedure. In this particular operation there is the possibility that the patient will have anesthesia of his face in the area of the surgery (meaning that the face will feel numb). Another possible side effect is a weakening of the chewing muscles on the operated side. (Of course, the patient would be advised of such surgical side effects prior to the operation. It is up to him to weigh the benefits and risks with the help of his physician before deciding to undergo the procedure. Most tic douloureux victims are willing to exchange their pain for muscle numbness or weakness.)

A surgical procedure for chronic-pain patients suffering from back pain is a disc operation. Diseased discs either can be fixed, partially removed, or fully removed. In many cases these procedures reduce or totally alleviate the pain.

Nerve Blocks

If the offending agent in the life of the chronic-pain patient is an injured nerve, a block of this nerve may be recommended by the pain-clinic staff. Nerve blocks are procedures during which an anesthesiologist injects a local anesthetic into a nerve to cut off its function. If its energy is cut, the nerve message is interrupted and does not reach the brain.

Nerve blocks also can be used as a diagnostic tool. If the staff is unsure which nerve or group of nerves is causing the patient's pain, an anesthesiologist may be called in. On successive days, he will block different nerves with an anesthetic, until both he and the patient are certain of the locations. Further treatment at this point may be either to continue blocking the offending nerve or to perform surgery—an incision or excision of the nerve so that its energy source is permanently cut off.

Electrical Stimulators

Electrical stimulators are devices used by pain clinics and physical therapists and by some private physicians to help combat pain by interrupting pain-nerve messages. Some of these devices are transcutaneous (across the skin) and some are implanted under the skin. At one pain clinic the devices have been successful with about 40 percent of the patients who have tried them but success depends on the type of pain.

The transcutaneous electrical stimulator merely applies a low voltage current between two electrodes on the skin. The implanted electrical stimulator is composed of a radio transmitter (a small plastic circle that sends impulses through the skin to a receiver that is taped to the lower back) and a power pack. The transmitter sends impulses to the receiver; the impulses block incoming pain messages traveling along the spinal cord. The power pack (which is about the size and shape of a cigarette pack and can be tucked away in a shirt pocket) sends electrical impulses to the transmitter. Patients who have used this device successfully say that they feel a pleasant, warm, tingling sensation. Others find the stimulator's sensation irritating.

Electrical stimulators are also designed so that the receiver component can be implanted in the back or even in the brain, where the effect is thought to be more potent.

In some pain clinics, the stimulator, a prescription item, is used as adjunctive therapy, rather than as a single treatment. If it is effective, it may be continuously worn by the patient, even when he sleeps.

Psychotherapy

Individual psychotherapy may offer support or employ supportive measures, or it may seek to find the source of problems by using a variety of techniques. These therapies help both the professional and the patient to explore the patient's personality and behavior patterns, to determine how chronic pain fits into his life, and to define and measure his emotional needs. Psychotherapy also seeks to help the patient find solutions to his problem by revealing his personality traits and guiding him toward insights about his flaws and strengths.

Group Therapy

Group therapy is a treatment technique that utilizes the dynamics of group interaction to achieve its ends: therapy and treatment for the patients in the group.

What are group dynamics? They include the reaction of individuals to one another in a group, role playing by the individual group members, the assumption of the leadership role by someone in the group and how this occurs, how followers react to the leader, and how each individual responds to the questions or statements of the other members of the group.

Individual members of groups learn from one another by seeing how they look and sound to other people. A group leader can be designated to act as a "facilitator of group dynamics." The group leader may be a psychiatrist, a licensed therapist, a social worker, or a member of the group.

In a pain clinic, group therapy deals with not only the responses and actions of individuals while they are in session together (usually for a one hour session each day), but it also includes all the interactions among patients on the ward. In pain clinics, chronic-pain patients eat together, take their recommended exercise therapy together, make their own beds, visit the nurses' station together to receive their medication, and talk to one another whenever they meet on the ward. They are continually interacting with one another, testing their behavior on these intimate strangers who in some ways share their pain. A comraderie develops among the patients and with it an understanding of how their fellow patients suffer. All this communication and interaction is therapy. It helps chronic-pain patients to readjust their thinking. They see what being ill and acting ill does to each of them, and they see how other people cope with being in pain. They learn that their method of handling pain is not the only way, and they learn that they are not the only people in the world who suffer from pain. This realization alone is therapeutic.

In an actual group session there are from five to fifteen people who participate in the discussion. If there are less than five people in the group, significant group dynamics won't take place; the group is too small for effective interaction to occur. With more than fifteen people, the group is too large for effective action; some members of the group will be lost in the crowd.

According to group theory, groups are considered to be either *heterogeneous,* made up of different types of members with basically different goals for therapy (such as a group of people waiting at a corner for a bus), or *homogeneous,* a group of people who have banded together for a common purpose (a group of conventioners waiting on a corner for a chartered bus to take them to a lecture hall for a continuing medical education session). Depending on whether the group is heterogeneous or homogeneous, group dynamics will occur at different rates and can be detrimental or beneficial to the individuals in the group.

Sometimes no significant dynamics occur, particularly in a heterogeneous group. The group of people who meet for therapy in a pain clinic is homogeneous; the patients have similar goals (relief of pain), and their interactions tend to be beneficial. They encourage one another when a good behavior is displayed, they criticize those members who are acting inappropriately and are possibly contributing to the continuation of their pain. How does this happen?

In the group setting an individual is more likely to air inner feelings that he may be too embarrassed to reveal on a one-to-one basis with a therapist. The group provides a support structure. The group also allows its member to see themselves as pain patients as they look at and listen to others who have pain complaints similar to their own. By comparing his behavior to others, a chronic-pain patient can see how he might help himself improve or recover.

In addition, group therapy is a useful diagnostic tool for some therapists. The interactions within a group sometimes will cause its members to physically arrange themselves into two groups: the copers—who freely admit to depression, anxiety, and other problems that their pain is causing them—on one side; the exaggerators—who refuse to admit to any of these problems, though depression or anxiety may be obvious from their outward appearance—on the other side.

The therapist might also be able to pinpoint exaggerators in a group therapy session by the way they talk about themselves. Exaggerators have a tendency to dwell on the severity of their symptoms and the degree of their incapacitation, and they try to compete with one another as to who has a greater amount of pain. Knowing which patient is a coper and which is an exaggerator helps the pain-clinic staff devise more effective treatment regimens.

Some deep-seated feelings are often brought out during a pain-clinic group-therapy session—particularly feelings of hopelessness, helplessness, and worthlessness. Patients feel a degree of security in a group and are able to express these feelings in the presence of others who can respond with empathy—something that few people will do for them in their everyday lives outside the clinic setting.

Finally, group sessions help patients ventilate their anger (an emotion that can contribute to tension). The anger may be directed at the doctors who failed them, who didn't believe in their pain, or it may be directed at a family member who has forsaken them. Chronic-pain patients also bottle up anger against people they perceive as controlling their lives, people on whom they are dependent and to whom they are now obligated. They may also be angry at themselves for having gotten into the position of being dependent, or for somehow having brought the pain on themselves. Ventilating anger also is therapeutic; it can release tension and is also a part of the attitude change that pain clinics seek.

Family Therapy

Family therapy, which emerged in the mid-1950s, is a relatively new branch of psychotherapy.

At that time, psychiatrists and psychologists decided to examine a phenomenon they saw occurring in some of the relatives of their patients. As soon as a patient appeared to improve, his relatives, rather than acting grateful or relieved, were suspicious and almost unhappy with the improvement. The families sought to pull the patient out of treatment or in some other way to undermine subtly the benefits the therapist was achieving. A good example of this phenomenon is the adolescent who, having achieved some success on a diet prescribed by her physician and vocally urged on by her mother, is suddenly told by her mother that she is too thin and that she should start eating more—even though the girl has not yet reached her weight goal.

As in groups, there is a system of dynamics or interaction that occurs within families. Each person in the family has a role and has power that goes with the role. Members of families interact with one another by wielding their power, mostly to maintain their power or their position in the family.

Thus psychiatrists and their colleagues have surmised that if one member of a family is emotionally or mentally ill, the illness probably has had an effect on other members of the family, too. Therefore, it would not be productive to treat the person with the problem without also treating the relatives who will be instrumental in either helping him recover or in prolonging his illness. In other words, not only is the patient sick but his family may be sick as well, and in order for the patient to regain his health, the family unit must also regain its health.

For example, if an adult, an exaggerator-type pain patient, has to move back in with his mother to receive the kind of care he needs, his mother may enjoy assuming the role of "mother" again—after having relinquished it when her child grew up and moved out of the house to be on his own. The mother might undermine the effects of therapy by keeping her child in bed, providing for his every whim, even though the therapist suggested that the patient move around as much as possible and stay out of bed until it was time to go to sleep.

A family therapist would call the mother into therapy with her son to discuss why she is keeping her son in bed, to help her explore her motives, and to show her why it is necessary that her son move about the house. Once the mother understands that her efforts to keep him dependent and at home are detrimental to his health, she can perhaps learn to let go and to help her son on the road to recovery.

Occupational Therapy

Occupational therapy aims to provide patients with marketable skills that accommodate the reduced abilities of the chronic-pain patient: if a warehouseman experiences chronic pain due to an injury from lifting a heavy load the wrong way, the occupational therapist can teach him the proper way to lift lighter loads, or the warehouseman might learn to do an entirely different job but one that he can use in his current place of employment; for example, he might learn to be an inventory clerk.

Such therapy works in two ways. Not only does the patient learn a skill to use back at his place of work that will help him to maintain himself economically, but the therapy also gives him confidence about his abilities (and perhaps about his ability to conquer pain). By providing new skills, occupational therapy reduces a patient's anxiety about what the future holds when he is no longer able to return to his old job. It gives him direction and something to focus on apart from his present incapacity.

Behavior Modification

Behavior modification is a way of changing behavior (what you do) with a system of rewards for good behavior, to encourage it to continue, and another system of punishments for bad behavior, to discourage its repetition. The cause for the action is not examined—only the action itself. Behavior modification for chronic-pain patients will be discussed more thoroughly in Chapter 8.

Biofeedback

Biofeedback once was considered a counterculture fad, a part of the meditation movement that promised to bring its advocates nirvana or inner peace by helping them to achieve their "alpha state," a restful state somewhere between consciousness and sleep.

The focus has changed away from alpha brain waves—and now medical investigators have adapted biofeedback as a mechanism for teaching people a new awareness of their body and the way it works as a means of achieving something more tangible than inner peace—relaxation and/or health. For example, by using the biofeedback machine you can become aware that a particular event, mood, thought, or person makes you tense (and tension, as you know, contributes to spasms and pain), and then you can learn to avoid it.

Biofeedback machines (which look like a stack of stereo components complete with knobs, swaying needles, and dials) measure energy output from muscles and body temperature. The electromyographic biofeedback machine, with the use of a computer and electrodes attached to specific muscles or critical temperature or pulse points, can teach the user to control certain physiological processes. The user can see what is going on in his body, how it is reacting, by looking at either an instantaneous display, a graphic representation, or an average activity over a period of time, depending on the model of machine in use.

Biofeedback has been found useful in the reduction of pain that is caused by spasms, migraine headaches, and tension. How exactly does biofeedback work?

Some experts suggest that pain is controlled by or reduced because of a distraction element, or because the patient has a sense of control over the pain, or as the result of hypnotic-like suggestion from an instructor. Others believe that biofeedback acts as a teaching mechanism: showing a person on a graph or ticker tape what is happening in his body at the moment it happens, he can learn to avoid a particular action that is causing him pain; he learns how to manipulate the pain by manipulating the graph.

For example, if the biofeedback's electrodes are placed on his temples and he clenches his jaws, he actually will see a rise in the tension of his muscles, graphically represented by a meter.

Therefore, if electrodes are attached to the point where a low-back-pain patient feels pain and he watches that pain (as muscle tension) register on the graph, he should be able to reduce his discomfort—if it is caused by tension—by making a conscious effort to relax. While watching the biofeedback display screen, he can try various methods of relaxing until he sees the meter reading drop. This drop should correspond with a reduction in pain.

Some researchers suggest that the reduction in pain may be due more to a "mental calm" than a reduction in muscle spasm.

This mental calm, they say, comes from the feeling that he has mastered his environment, or more important, that he has come to know and master his body and its responses.

Victims of chronic pain often feel as if they have been robbed, both of good health and freedom from pain. They also feel as if they no longer are in control of their lives—certainly an uncomfortable feeling. Biofeedback machines teach them to take control again and in that process help them help themselves to reduce their pain.

(You can purchase your own biofeedback machine and teach yourself to relax at home. For the appropriate type of machine and training, your physician should be consulted.)

Hypnosis

Hypnosis is an old treatment in the chronic-pain field and has been applied "scientifically" for a variety of other problems for nearly three centuries.

Dr. Friedrich Anton Mesmer, an Austrian physician, first used his system of suggestion and relaxation to control and influence his patients. His patients thus were "mesmerized." To add to the effect, electrical current was applied to patients.

Hypnosis has been accepted for a long time as a valid tool in psychotherapy, but its use as an analgesic is, along with many of the techniques mentioned in this chapter, new to the field of pain research and relief. Again, as with biofeedback, hypnosis functions primarily as a tool to help the patient focus his attention away from his pain or his symptoms of pain.

Though not all people can be hypnotized, the climate for hypnotism is better and more apt to produce results if a physician can establish a rapport with his patients. Basically, hypnotism plays on the mind's ability to be therapeutic to itself, such as our ability to forget painfully embarrassing incidents or change them into incidents at which we can laugh.

Hypnotism is essentially an altered state of awareness, one in which the patient is able to disassociate himself from his environment, either at the suggestion of the hypnotist or at the patient's own suggestion (autohypnosis), and concentrate on subjects or perceptions that need to be altered. The ability to concentrate this deeply varies among individuals, but it is most likely to be found in people who are open to the suggestion that there *are* several different states of consciousness. Some investigators have found that people who take naps during the day or who are able to fall asleep quickly at night or whenever they want to are likely to be good subjects for hypnosis.

A pain patient undergoing hypnosis receives a suggestion from the hypnotist to imagine that he is performing some other activity; for example, he is told that instead of sitting in the hypnotist's chair, he is taking a train ride through some pretty countryside. Though the patient's central nervous system may be receiving pain messages, his perception and reception of the messages are diverted. Because of the hypnotic suggestion, the patient is absorbed in the mental image of his pleasant train ride; he feels the rhythm of the train swaying against his body—at least he imagines that he does. This enjoyable experience suppresses the pain perception, as the train ride takes center stage in the patient's state of consciousness.

The hypnotist also can plant pain-killing suggestions in patients who are unable to achieve the trancelike state required to push aside all perception of pain. Some researchers have found that these posthypnotic suggestions may help make the pain tolerable. Other researchers believe that hypnosis merely creates a relaxed and trusting atmosphere between patient and therapist, which helps the patient to reduce his anxiety, tension, and some of his pain. It also helps the patient to think about his pain in a new way—to realize that pain exists only if it is perceived. If the patient can learn to modify or divert his perceptions, the impact of pain upon its victim will be altered even though the stimulus that produces it still endures.

Again, as with biofeedback, you can be taught how to use hypnosis to your advantage, to achieve a peaceful and/or relaxed state, a state that counteracts pain. However, its use in chronic pain is limited.

Acupuncture

Acupuncture once was scoffed at by Western scientists as a primitive Eastern folk remedy, on a par with an American Indian medicine man shaking a rattle to ward off evil spirits, i.e., merely hypnotic-like suggestion. Just as the medicine man's techniques are better understood by mental health professionals, so acupuncture may now be seen to have some use.

Acupuncture uses a body chart of trigger points and a series of needles. These needles are twisted or twirled in a certain manner at the trigger points. Depending on the disease and on the chronic-pain location, a different number of needles will be twisted in different trigger spots on the body. Some needles are left in the trigger points over a period of time, twirled anywhere from ten or twenty minutes, and then removed.

Scientists speculate that acupuncture may have an effect on the chronic pain of some patients because it stimulates certain nerve pathways to send messages to the brain counteracting the pain messages. Acupuncture also may stimulate circulation to parts of the body that have been damaged by the effects of poor circulation, a situation that often can cause pain.

In addition, acupuncture may have a placebo effect; that is, if the patient believes that the technique will help him, it *will* help him. Recent research suggests it may work by stimulating the production of a morphine-like chemical in the body.

Physical Therapy

Physical therapy is an important treatment for almost all chronic-pain patients. Most chronic-pain patients tend to avoid any activity in order not to aggravate a painful spot. However muscles that are not used get stiff and can cause additional pain when the patient finally attempts to use them again. For these people walking alone may be good therapy. Some pain patients undergo recommended operations and need physical therapy following the surgery in order to regain the use of a limb.

For some patients the physical therapy in the pain clinic is simple. It also is relaxing. Physical therapy can take place in a small room with just one person and the therapist or it can be a group activity. In the group setting it usually is set to music.

The therapy may consist of stretching motions to limber unused tendons and muscles. These movements include raising an arm up and down or moving the neck from side to side. The therapy can include bending motions that use more than one set of muscles, such as bending from the waist with the hands dangling to the toes, then straightening the torso and bending backwards.

Because physical therapy is something that you can do at home to help yourself cope with pain, we are including a list of exercises that, when done on a daily basis, constitute a useful exercise program for most pain patients. The exercises help strengthen and stretch muscles throughout the body.

A warning: it is common to experience some muscle guarding (limitation of use) or spasms in the area of pain. This is the body's natural reaction to pain. You feel pain and you want to avoid it, so you protect yourself by not moving your muscles. This limitation of motion leads to a decreased ability to move at will and this leads to more pain. Therefore it is necessary to keep joints moving freely to help decrease muscle guarding.

The following are some exercises used at a major teaching hospital's Pain Treatment Center. Check with your own physician prior to utilizing any of them. They are used primarily for back pain.

Exercises

Easy

STANDING:

Upper Extremities: 10 times each

(1) Stretch arms straight overhead, one at a time.
(2) Stretch arms straight forward, one at a time.
(3) Shrug shoulders, hold a few seconds, relax.
(4) Raise arms to shoulder level, elbows bent; bring elbows backward, squeezing shoulder blades together; then stretch arms across front of body.
(5) Do "swimming" strokes, making big circles with arms first forward, then backward.

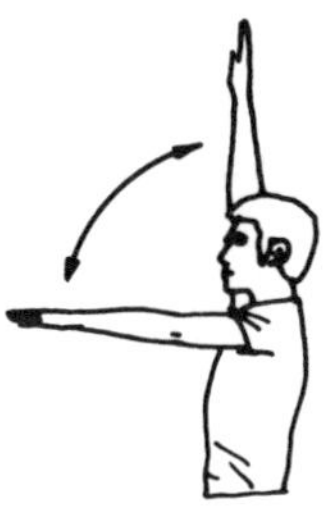
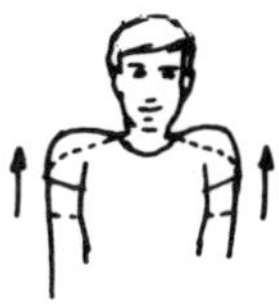
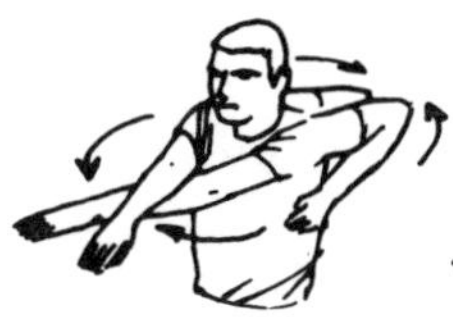
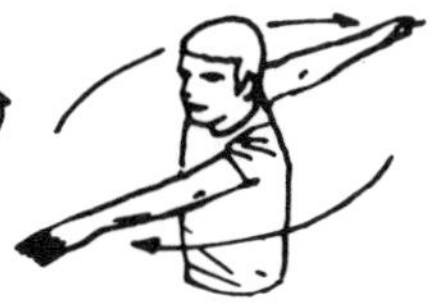

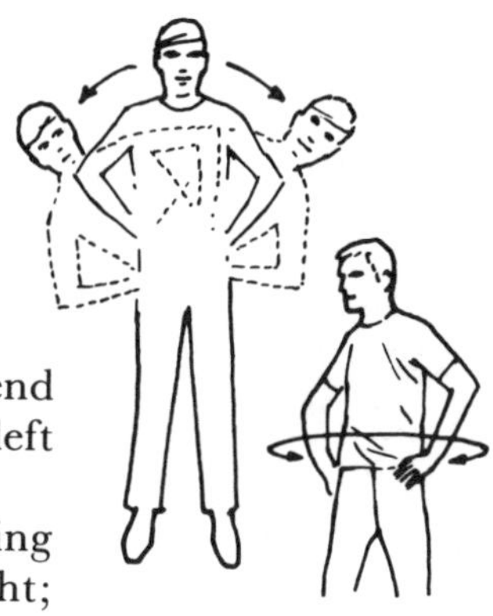

Trunk Muscles: 10 times each

(1) Stand with feet slightly apart; bend from waist to right side, then to left side. (Do not bend forward.)
(2) Keep hips and lower extremities facing forward; rotate upper trunk to right; then to left.

Lower Extremities: 10 times each

(1) Put one leg forward, keeping heels on floor; bend front knee (should feel stretching in back calf muscle).
(2) March in place (at least two minutes).

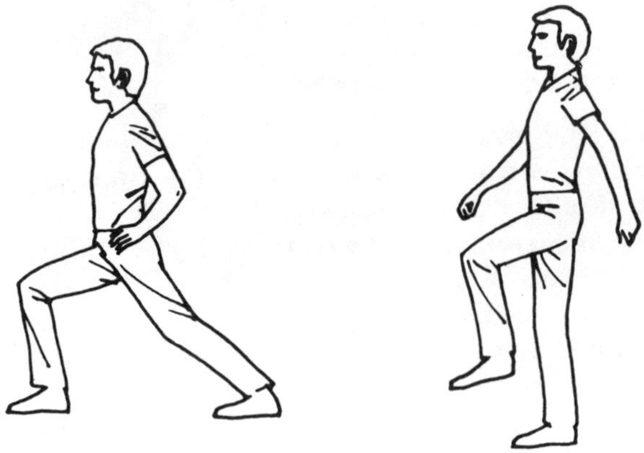

SITTING:

Lower Extremities: 10 times each

(1) Pull one knee up toward chest, then straighten leg; hold, and relax.
(2) Slide to edge of chair; pull both knees up toward chest, hold, and relax. (Do not lean on back of chair.)
(3) Sitting on edge of chair, bend forward bringing arms through knees to touch floor.
(4) Lift both feet off floor; make circles with ankles.

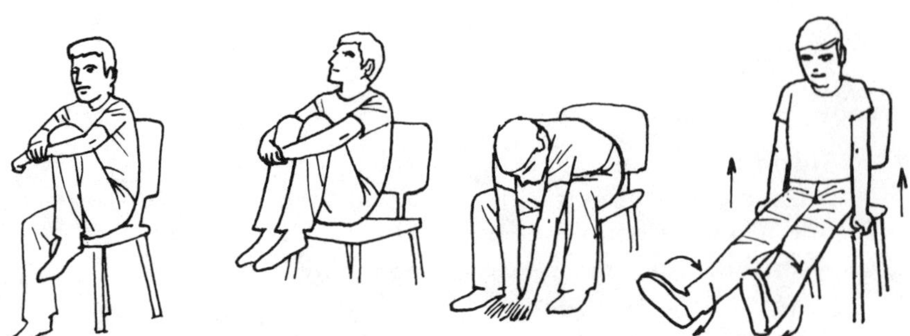

Neck Exercises: 10 times each

(1) Clasp hands in back of head, push head back into hands (isometric contraction), hold, and relax.
(2) Touch chin to chest and roll shoulders forward, hold, and relax (feel stretching in back of neck).
(3) Look straight ahead; bend head toward shoulder to right, then left. (Do not bring shoulder toward ear.)
(4) Turn head clockwise, then counterclockwise, hold, and relax.

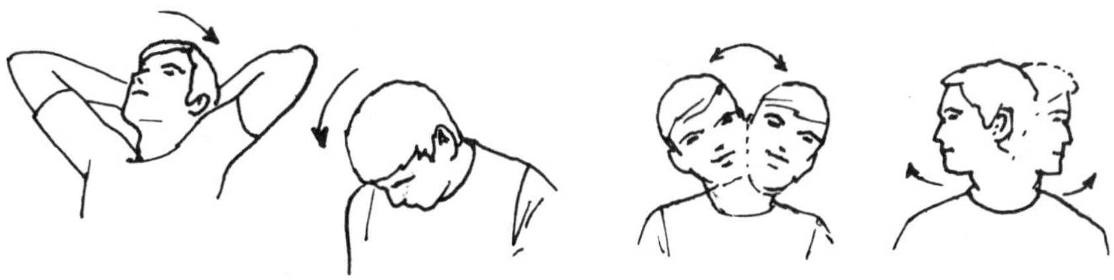

FOR THOSE WHO CAN SIT ON FLOOR: 5 times

Sit in long sitting position, legs out in front with knees straight; bend trunk forward and try to touch toes with hands.

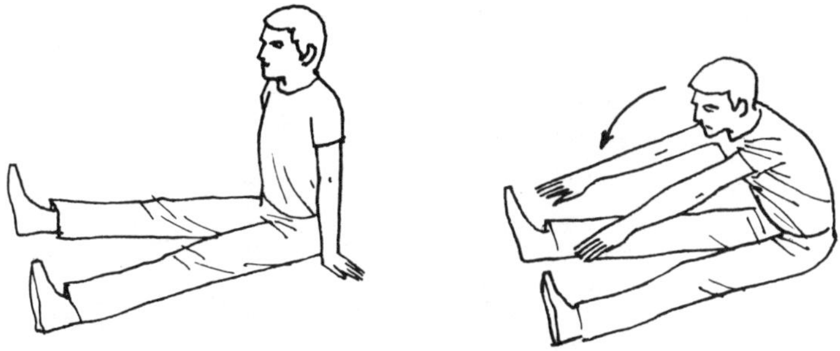

Advanced

Here are some more difficult exercises. They can be used as part of a prevention program or as a way out of pain. Weak backs and unexercised muscles are vulnerable to pain. These exercises will strengthen the muscles and keep the body limber.

1. *Pelvic tilt*

   a. Begin by lying on your back with knees bent.
   b. Tighten stomach muscles and flatten lower back against table, thus tipping pelvis backward; hold to count of 3 and relax.
   c. Repeat 20 times.

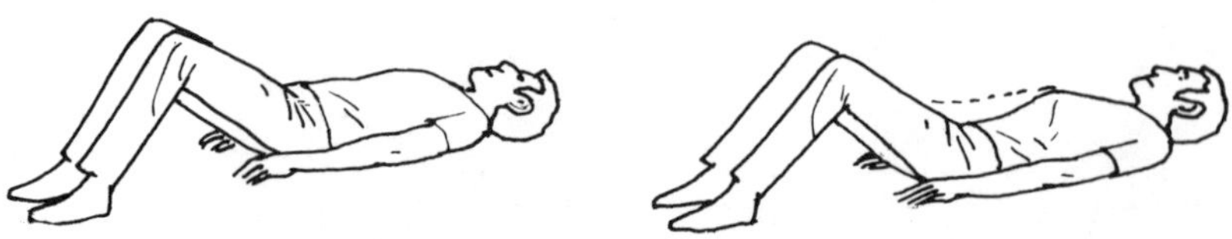

2. *Knees to chest*

   a. Begin by lying on your back with knees bent.
   b. Bend one knee toward shoulder as far as possible and return to original position.
   c. Alternate legs.
   d. Repeat 10 times. Do 2 sets.

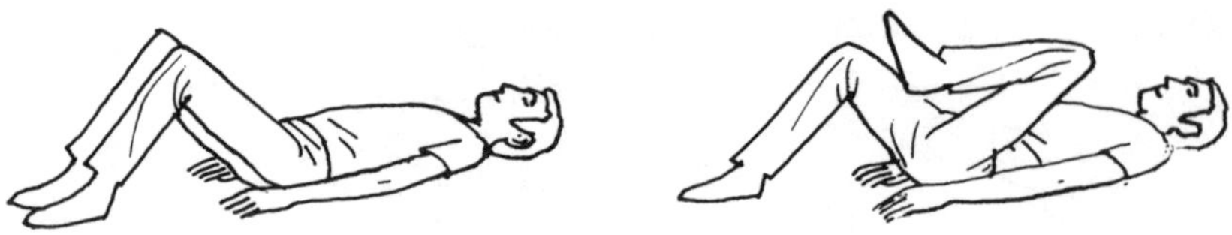

3. *Modified bicycle*

   a. Begin by lying on your back with knees bent.
   b. Bend one knee toward chest, then straighten knee as far as possible and lower, keeping knee straight. *Keep opposite knee bent.*
   c. Alternate legs.
   d. Repeat 10 times. Do 2 sets.

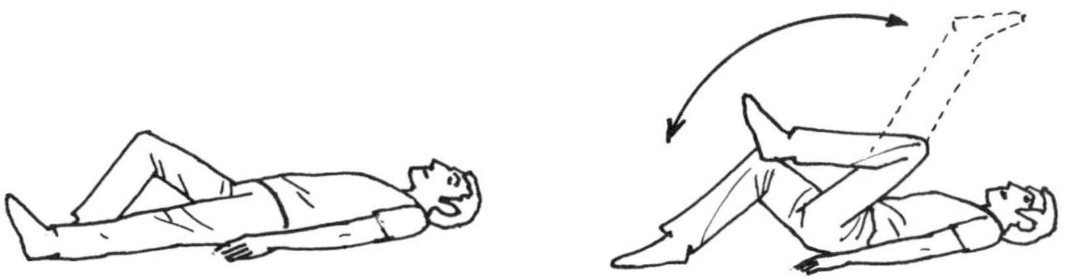

4. *Sit-ups*

   a. Begin by lying on your back with knees bent and feet hooked under a heavy object.
   b. Hold arms straight ahead about 20 inches off the floor.
   c. Keeping arms straight, roll chin to chest and sit up as far as possible; try to roll into a ball.
   d. Return to original position slowly, keeping chin to chest.
   e. Repeat 10 times. Do 2 sets.

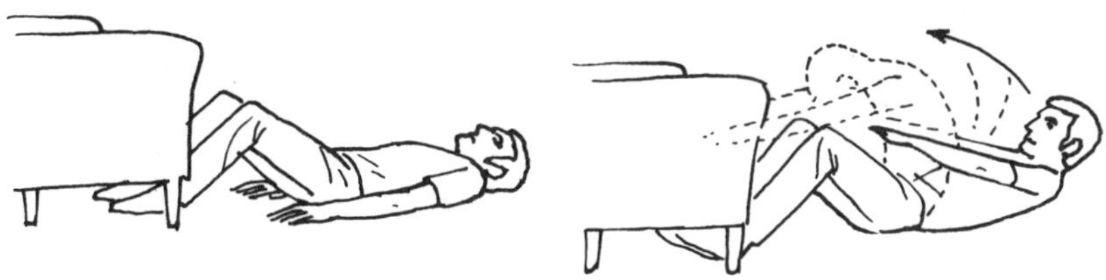

5. *Cat's back*

   a. Begin on hands and knees.
   b. Arch upper back like a cat.
   c. Bend one knee to chest; then kick the leg back, keeping knee straight and leg parallel to floor; bend knee to chest again and return to original position.
   d. Alternate legs.
   e. Repeat 10 times with each leg. Do 2 sets.

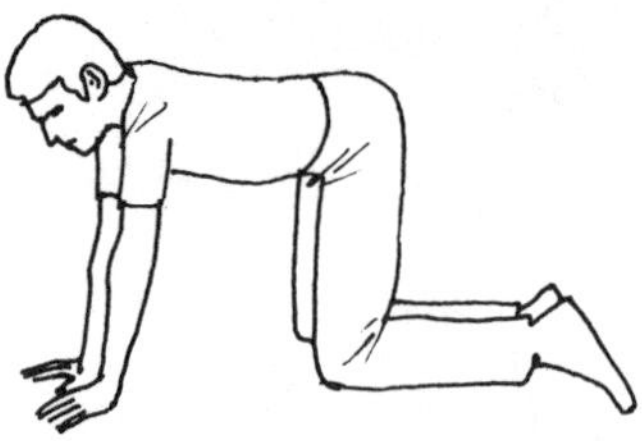

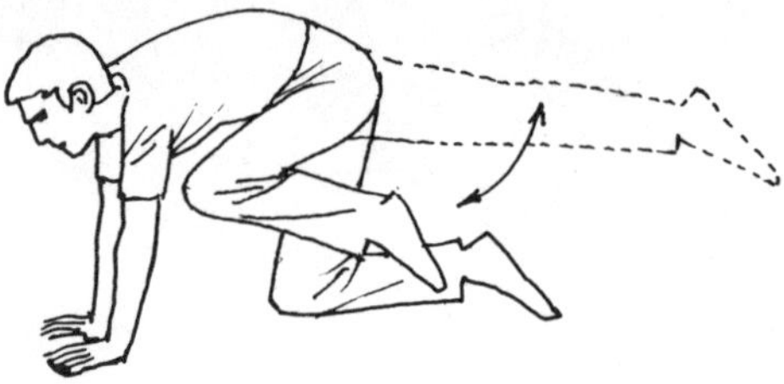

6. *Kneel and stretch*

   a. Begin on hands and knees.
   b. Then sit back so that buttocks are resting on heels.
   c. Reach arms forward as far as possible with forehead resting on floor; keep buttocks on heels.
   d. Repeat 10 times. Do 2 sets.

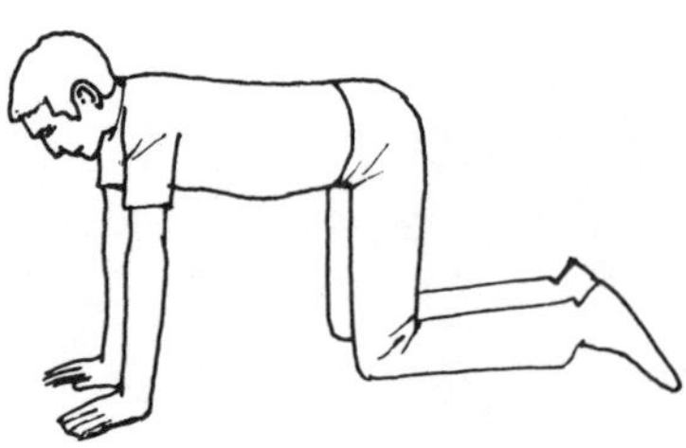

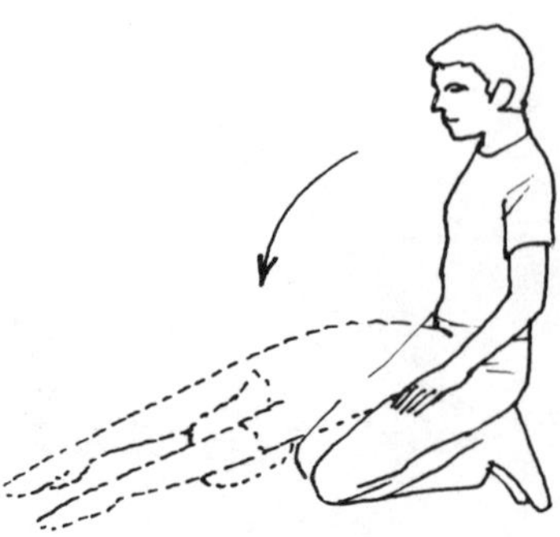

7. *Bridging*

a. Begin by lying on your back with knees bent.
b. Lift hips and buttocks off floor.
c. Hold.
d. Return to starting position.
e. Repeat 10 times.

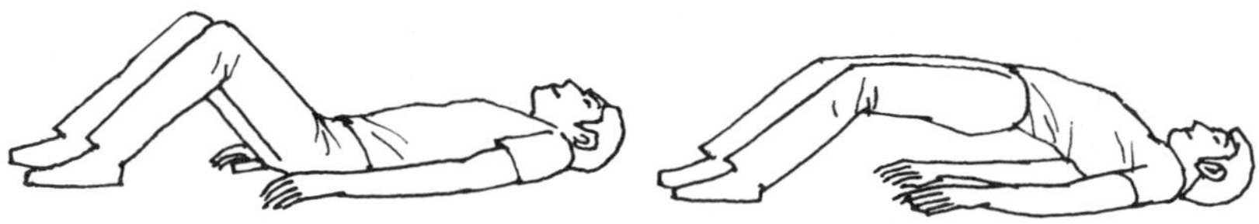

8. *Bobbing*

a. Sit on the edge of a chair that is braced against a wall.
b. Fold forearms across chest with hands hooked in the crooks of elbows.
c. Place feet flat on floor with knees well apart.
d. Put head down; drop elbows as far between legs as possible.
e. Bob toward floor 5 times, sit up, and repeat 5 times.
f. Do not drag arms down front of legs.

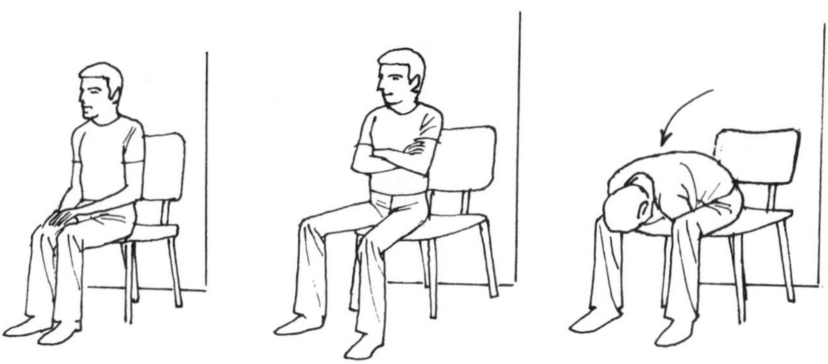

Taking care of your back

When standing for long periods of time, put one foot up on footstool.

Sleep best on side with both knees bent, or on back with two pillows under the knees. Avoid sleeping on the stomach.

Do not maintain any one position for any length of time; keep moving, but not necessarily vigorously.

When sitting, keep whole back supported, especially when driving.

It may help to have a small pillow in the small of the back.

Do not lift any objects weighing over 3 pounds. Do necessary lifting with the *legs;* bend knees to reach the floor, not waist.

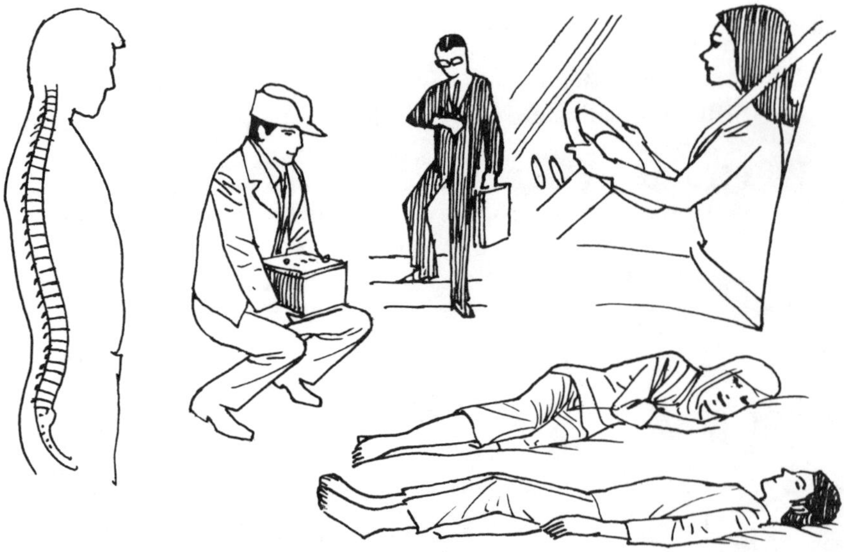

7
Pain Clinics and What They Can Do for You

No *one* of the therapies we have discussed (most are available in a physician's office or hospital medical center) may be the best approach to chronic pain. A combination of therapies has been found to be useful in a number of cases. The varied approach is offered at the multidisciplinary pain-treatment center. Multidisciplinary means that many specialists are on hand and many more are available for consulation for each chronic-pain patient. In this era of specialists, who sometimes treat diseases just of the hand or the foot or a single organ, the multidisciplinary team assures that the whole person will be treated. John Bonica, M.D., set up the first multidisciplinary pain-treatment center in the state of Washington, at University Hospital in Seattle, twenty-five years ago and pioneered many of the therapies still in use today.

The multidisciplinary team that staffs a pain-treatment center can be composed of a neurologist, a neurosurgeon, an orthopedic surgeon, a psychiatrist, a dentist, a radiologist, an ophthalmologist, an otolaryngologist, a pharmacologist, a social worker, a psychiatric nurse, a psychologist, a physical therapist, an internist, an occupational therapist, and maybe even a scientist working on a research grant. One pain clinic in New York has nineteen different specialists available for consultation.

A pain clinic associated with a hospital can usually consult with the medical staff of the hospital if the regular staff of the clinic is baffled by a particular pain problem or pain patient.

The multidisciplinary staff works together as a team. The team concept of medical care is especially successful with chronic-pain patients who not only present complex physical problems but who suffer from either depression or anxiety and who may respond to one kind of health professional and not another. Team members in a pain clinic work together as a detective agency and as a support mechanism for the patient (and with difficult cases, as support for each other as they pursue their goal of helping the patient at any cost).

Each member of the team who examines a chronic-pain patient meets with the other members to report his findings, and then the team pools its information and insights in order to come to a consensus on the patient's therapy. It is important that the chronic-pain patient receive this type of evaluation. The possibility of an obscure disease or a personality disorder being overlooked, or of patient/physician incompatability interfering with the diagnosis and treatment, are greatly reduced.

When a chronic-pain patient visits one specialist, he receives the benefit of that person's skills in his specialty. Yet his pain may not fall within the realm of the specialist's specific knowledge and skills. With the multidisciplinary team, many specialists are available to cross-check findings, and they have a better chance of relieving pain by discovering its cause than does a single doctor. Utilizing its group knowledge, the team can function somewhat like a computer, receiving information and using it to formulate a solution—a solution that they can suggest to the patient to help him for his own goal or goals for therapy.

Who are these people who make up the multidisciplinary team? A typical team might consist of a head nurse, a nurse, a physician's assistant, a social worker, a psychiatrist, a physical therapist, an anesthesiologist, a psychologist, a nursing administrator, an orthopedic surgeon, a technician, and a neurosurgeon.

The *neurosurgeon* is a physician who specializes in correcting diseases, injuries, or other problems related to the brain and nervous system. Brain surgery is rarely warranted in certain types of chronic pain; but if tumors press on nerve centers in the brain—these tumors must be removed. The majority of their work in chronic pain revolves around their skill and knowledge of the spinal cord and autonomic nervous system.

The *technician* operates the diagnostic equipment found in the pain-clinic setting; for example, the technician might be a member of the radiology department and therefore be specially trained to handle X-ray equipment. Other technicians specialize in the use of biofeedback machines or thermographic units. Though not a physician, the technician is a specialist too.

The *psychiatrist* is a physician who specializes in dealing with emotional problems and mental illness. The psychologist also specializes in these areas, but he is not a physician and therefore cannot prescribe drugs. The psychologist, however, is licensed to practice by a state board. One of the major roles of a psychiatrist or psychologist is to *listen* to the problems of the patients, to empathize with them, and to help the patient form his own solutions to his problems. How the psychiatrist or psychologist handles patients' therapy differs according to his philosophical leanings or the theory of psychology he had adopted (for example, Freudian, Jungian, Adlerian, reality, or paradoxical). However, many psychiatrists have found an eclectic approach to be most successful.

The *anesthesiologist* who is also a physician, is an authority on the characteristics of analgesic-type drugs and their effects on the body. Anesthesiologists frequently are called in to determine whether nerve blocks are the answer for a chronic-pain patient. One method that an anesthesiologist might use to determine whether a particular nerve is the culprit in chronic pain is to test an anesthetic on several different nerves. The test uses both an anesthetic and a placebo on a group of nerves. If the pain stops in one nerve with the anesthetic and not with the placebo (and doesn't stop with either substance in the remaining nerves) the anesthesiologist can be pretty sure he has found the offending nerve, which then becomes a candidate for a block.

A *social worker* follows close on the heels of the psychiatrist or psychologist. He is trained to investigate the home situation and its effect on the chronic-pain patient. The social worker evaluates the patient's family and offers a solution that allows the patient to smooth over strained relationships.

The *nursing staff* has the closest and most ongoing contact with the chronic-pain patient. The nursing administrator arranges his schedule, and the head nurse and nurses attend to his daily needs and wants. The nursing staff can report to the other specialists on the team any changes in personality, attitude, or behavior that they note, and that might be important to his recovery.

A physician's assistant is a licensed practitioner who can provide simple medical services, freeing up the specialists for more complicated medical tasks. On a pain-treatment ward the physician's assistant might take blood pressures, give injections, palpate sore spots, and report back to the team his impressions of the general health of the patient.

This is just a sampling of staff members on a pain-clinic team. Different combinations of different specialists and technicians may be available at the various pain clinics around the country. Whatever the combination, all the staff members work in concert to help you reach your therapy goals.

Establishing goals is a key undertaking at a pain clinic. If you just visit *a* doctor, his goal will be to stop your complaint of pain by using medication. If you visit *a* surgeon, he will be oriented toward a surgical solution, in order to remove the pain. If you are taking pills, your goal is to relieve the pain. But in the pain clinic, the goal is not necessarily the relief of pain. The goal could be change in attitudes, values, or lifestyle. The goal may be to withdraw you from drugs. This withdrawal may give you more relief in the long run than anything else you may have tried. Whatever the goal, it will not be established by you alone, or by doctors alone, but by a team of which you will be one of the members.

Because each chronic-pain patient suffers from pain in his own way, treatment plans and goals are individualized, tailored to specific needs and perhaps to specific pocketbooks. A treatment course can take anywhere from two weeks to several months to execute and may have to be repeated at another point in time, depending on the severity of the problem. The cost can vary according to whether or not the plan is carried out on an inpatient or outpatient basis. For example, if an operation is called for, treatment plus recuperation and follow-up therapy could take more than several months. Some people need to be readmitted two, three, or four times to a pain clinic in order to achieve their goal. Some may be helped on an inpatient basis with a one-week stay. Others may visit the clinic from their home base on a daily basis for a month. (All these factors contribute to cost.)

A patient may be striving to reach more than one goal. Some patients may set a goal of completing a therapy suggested by the team; some may set an occupational goal for themselves—perhaps learning to tolerate the pain to the point where they can return to work or get a different job to accommodate the limitations imposed on them by their pain.

In some eyes the goal may be minimal, such as setting a recreational goal that you will attend one of every three family outings. The goal may be a personal one, such as reestablishing a relationship with a family member alienated during the worst of the chronic-pain period in your life.

No one, however, is forced to participate in those recommended portions of the program of the pain clinic that lead to these goals. The staff will explain to you though that failure to participate in suggested portions of the activities can, and probably will, lead to failure in the search for pain relief. Becoming a patient at a pain clinic means making a commitment to your treatment. You cannot just be a receiver of care, prescriptions, or operations at a pain clinic. You must be an active participant in your treatment plan. You can't reach your goal by sitting on the sidelines.

How do you become a patient at a pain-treatment clinic? The easiest route is through referral by your family physician to a pain clinic in your area. If possible, you then can be seen on an outpatient basis and will be able to cut the cost by living at home (only if surgery has been ruled out, of course). If you live too far to commute, it is possible to be hospitalized in a clinic, if the clinic has the bed space. Some clinics are associated with teaching hospitals; in these cases, you may be hospitalized in a nearby institution.

Being referred to a pain clinic does not necessarily mean that you will become a patient at one. Most clinics are small and bed space is tight. You probably will be interviewed before being taken on.

If you are not placed on a waiting list, the next step before admission to a clinic (in some treatment centers) is a screening examination. Different pain clinics use different screening mechanisms to determine what type of patient they are dealing with. The results from these tests are also used to determine treatment goals and therapy progress. Treatment plans are then individualized.

In the multidisciplinary pain clinics all parts of the proffered program are voluntary. No one is forced to do anything he does not want to do; however, patients who don't fully participate rarely obtain optimal benefits.

While you are participating in therapy that includes any of the previously listed methods, you also will be partaking of a substantial amount of physical activity, activity that will help to improve your overall physical fitness as well as your attitude about the limitations that you have placed on yourself because of the pain. You probably will be walking, climbing stairs, sitting, standing, doing almost anything but stewing about the life of pain you have lead.

As part of your therapy in many pain clinics, you will not be allowed to talk about your pain to anyone anywhere except in scheduled therapy sessions. Nurses and other ward personnel are aware of this restriction and will not make conversation with you on the subject of pain. Your verbalization of your pain on the ward will be limited to answering the questions of the physician making rounds or the nurse inquiring about your general health during the day.

You will be asked to do many things despite your complaints of pain. If, for example, you say you cannot walk to the bathroom because of the pain in your legs, the nurse may ask you to take a few steps each day toward the bathroom until you are able to walk there unassisted and without prodding.

Life on the ward will not be luxurious. Your whims will not be catered to, particularly those pertaining to medication. If you are used to swallowing a pill when you feel the pain coming on, you will be forced to do without the pain-killers on the ward. You will not be given pain-killers on demand, rather you will receive medication from the staff when they deem it advisable.

You may have visitors, family or friends, but they too will be instructed not to cater to you. They will be instructed not to discuss your pain with you, nor will you be allowed to discuss your treatment with them. This is all part of a treatment program that serves to refocus your thinking. Pain is banished as much as possible from your world—not only physically, when possible, but also psychically.

Remember, chronic pain is not an emergency. Treating chronic pain takes time, just as the chronic pain took time to erode part of your life. Treatment comes after careful diagnosis, and relief comes only with a change in your attitude. As a patient in a pain-treatment clinic, you must be motivated, you must be certain that you want to get well. Then the pain clinic can work for you and can help you master your pain.

Ultimately the time it takes to conquer chronic pain or adjust to the pain so that you can function as you want to is up to you and to your attitude: no single thing, not the surgeon's knife, not a single magical pill, not a flow of kind words, will help you manage or eliminate your pain.

In the pain clinic the treatment for intractable pain begins with belief and trust. The staff proceeds from the belief that all patients who come to them for help are in pain, and the pain is not just "in their heads." In this way the staff elicits a sense of trust from the patients. Trust is an enormous help when any kind of care is given, but it is particularly useful when dealing with chronic-pain patients who often feel as though they've been left along medicine's highway without a friend. With trust, patients are more apt to participate in those recommended treatments that otherwise might have seemed frightening or overwhelming.

Treatments are tailor-made in the pain clinics. No one treatment or combination of therapies is exactly the same for every patient, just as no one's pain is the same as anyone else's.

Treatment ranges from simple withdrawal from drugs to highly complex surgery requiring skill and advanced equipment. All procedures, however, are aimed at treating the *disease* called chronic pain.

A Pain Victim's Odyssey

It may be helpful for you to see what it's like to be a victim of chronic pain—to seek help and to fail to find it. Sometimes the trail can end in disaster and financial ruin, or sometimes it can lead to the therapy that brings relief. The woman in the following account was fortunate, her quest ended at a pain clinic.

Harriet is twenty-four years old. She worked very hard for two years after high school to save enough money to put toward the entrance fee and tuition payments in a nursing program. Harriet's lifelong dream was to become a registered nurse, wear the profession's white uniform, and help sick people. Even as a child, when Harriet playacted, she was a nurse.

Harriet was like a whirlwind in her nursing program, running from class to class, working after school to keep up with the tuition payments, and trying to enjoy some sort of social life by accepting an occasional casual date on weekends. Harriet's only regret was that she had to live at home instead of in the dormitory with the other nursing students: the money she saved on room and board went for incidental school expenses.

Harriet's whirlwind came to a painful stop the day after she wore a brand new pair of crepe-sole nursing shoes that she had bought on sale. The shoes did not fit exactly right, but she liked how they looked. Harriet wore them all day on the ward, and they pinched and rubbed her feet until she developed several painful blisters. Even though she did not wear the shoes the next day to class and her blisters were all bandaged, her left foot continued to throb.

Harriet thought that she might have pulled a muscle from foolishly walking in tight shoes, and she tried to ignore the pain. But after a week the throbbing still had not disappeared, and she had to curtail her part-time job and her ward work because the pain made it difficult for her both to stand and to concentrate.

Several weeks later her foot was so painful that she could not wear stockings and was unable to put any weight on the toes of her left foot. She hobbled to classes as well as she could, but she found that going to classes was at best a waste of time: she could not listen to lectures, she could not concentrate, and she did not feel like taking notes. At worst, going to class was extremely trying and painful.

Harriet became even more determined to ignore the pain and asked a fellow student to accompany her to the student health clinic so that she could get a pair of crutches. She thought that with the aid of crutches she would be able to keep her weight off her painful foot and perhaps make it to classes without feeling exhausted from the pain. The friend said that she would help Harriet get the crutches, but she insisted that Harriet see a doctor in the student health service.

Harriet told the physician assigned to student health about her problem with her foot. At first the physician suspected that Harriet's pain was caused by thrombophlebitis, an inflammation of the major veins in the legs (during his last days in office, President Richard Nixon was afflicted with several painful bouts of thrombophlebitis that caused him to take rest periods during the day and keep his foot up on a stool.) The doctor ordered a phlebogram for Harriet. She spent several days in the hospital while she waited for the results. When the test came back, the results were negative.

Harriet told her doctor that lately she had been very depressed, and that she was feeling anxious that she would miss her final exams. She had even dreamed about missing them. She told the doctor that she was desperate, she wanted to get rid of the pain, not only because it hurt but even more because it prevented her from doing everything she wanted to do and felt needed to be done.

Although the doctor prescribed several potent narcotic painkillers and sleeping pills, Harriet's pain did not clear up and continued to interfere with her activity by making her immobile. After several weeks of observation in the student clinic, her condition had become so bad that water splashing on her thigh from a sponge bath was enough to cause her considerable pain.

The student health physician called in an orthopedic surgeon, who immediately gave Herriet a complete series of examinations. The surgeon could find nothing wrong in any of these tests, and she suggested that a psychiatric evaluation might be in order. She felt that Harriet might be overreacting to the pressures of schoolwork and the emotional stress of working on a ward for the first time.

The psychiatrist referred Harriet to a pain clinic that was near the school campus. The psychiatrist had an office there.

On her admission, the staff of the pain-treatment center asked Harriet a series of questions to determine how she felt in general and how she thought the pain altered her life-style.

The staff found Harriet to be a highly motivated young lady, one who had goals set for herself and was depressed becaused achieving them seemed to be so far in the future, when only a few months before they had seemed so close at hand. They also discovered that Harriet was angry with doctors—she thought that they did not believe that she was in pain. She did not trust them anymore because she felt that they did not trust her to be honest with them. She also was upset because she got the distinct feeling that the student health physician thought she was faking her pain to get attention or to get out of taking her final exams.

Harriet also was indulging in some self-pity, the staff decided. She was feeling sorry for herself because she believed she might never realize her dream of being a nurse. Most of all, Harriet was miserable. She was distressed by the pain and she was distressed because all the pills prescribed for her made her feel groggy and robbed of her ability to think sharply, a talent she considered to be one of her most precious possessions.

Harriet received a complete physical exam and filled out a medical history for the pain-center records.

The internist in charge of her physical looked at her legs several times and found that her left foot was mildly swollen (edema), mostly about the toes. Her left leg also seemed to be cooler to the touch than her lower right leg. When he tried to examine her left leg more closely, Harriet told him he was causing her a great deal of pain, sharp shooting pain. The internist then asked Harriet to stand up and place weight on both her legs equally. Harriet did this with difficulty. She could not fully extend her left knee. Otherwise, Harriet appeared to be a healthy young woman.

Because of the marked difference in temperature between her

lower left leg and her right one, the internist ordered a thermographic exam, in which, as explained in Chapter 5, areas of pain can be mapped out by their decreased temperature compared to normal tissue temperature. The thermograph showed that there was a generalized coldness from her foot to her calf in her left leg as compared to the right leg. The lower left leg was as much as two degrees centigrade cooler (an average temperature difference in positive findings in thermography). The thermographic map of the painful area suggested that there was some damage to a sympathetic nerve in her leg.

Harriet checked into the pain clinic as an inpatient. She agreed to follow the rules of the clinic and signed a "contract" with the staff regarding her participation. The physician in charge informed her about the possible sympathetic nerve damage, explaining in lay terms what it meant. He suggested that she try a lumbar sympathetic block (a block to nerves in the lower regions of the back). Harriet agreed.

The blocks were performed at the pain clinic by an anesthesiologist. Harriet had immediate relief from her pain.

When the effect of the block wore off and the pain returned, Harriet returned to the clinic. The pain clinic once again recommended a lumbar sympathetic block, which again was successful.

Following this procedure, the staff psychiatrist, anesthesiologist, internist, and social worker got together and discussed Harriet's case. They felt that Harriet would be a good candidate for a sympathectomy, a surgical severing of the nerve that was causing her pain (as shown by the success of blocking that nerve). Harriet had proved to be a motivated patient who had a good premorbid adjustment and who showed signs of trying to cope with and adjust to the pain, but was frustrated in her efforts.

After explaining the benefits and risks of the surgery to Harriet, the staff recommended that she have the operation. Harriet agreed. She had immediate relief from the pain and went on to finish her studies.

She returned to the pain clinic two years later for a follow-up study of her progress. The new thermograph showed that her lower left leg was a full 2.5 degrees warmer than it had been during her period of pain.

Since the operation and after receiving her degree, Harriet has worked as a registered nurse—a busy one who walks all day without discomfort. She also wears shoes that fit.

Not all patients who enter the pain clinic are as big a success story as Harriet. It is true that some people never receive complete relief from pain. In these cases, the staff continues to support them, and help them in every way they can to be active and to function to their fullest.

8
How You Can Help Yourself
Behavior Modification

One of the primary goals of a pain-treatment center is to change the patient's behavior with respect to his pain. Because the pain over time has slowly modified the patient's behavior—altered it—and has affected everything he does, the pain clinic staff must try to re-alter that behavior so that the pain is no longer the focus of the patient's life.

Behavior is the manner in which a person responds to his environment—when he is alone or among other people. Behavior modification is a system of altering behavior by a variety of means.

Operant (Skinnerian) conditioning is a form of behavior modification that is used in some clinics: if the behavior exhibited is considered desirable, a reward is given; when behavior that is undesirable is displayed, a punishment is given to discourage a repeat performance. In other words, an outside force, whoever is dispensing the rewards or punishments, is changing the behavior, rather than the patient changing his behavior solely on his own.

The classic experiment in instrumental (classical) conditioning involved Pavlov's dog, who was taught to salivate at the sound of a bell. Whenever the caged animal heard a bell, he was immediately given a piece of food. This action was repeated often enough so that the dog came to expect the food (expectation shown by salivation) whenever he heard a bell, wherever he was.

In the pain clinic, before a system of rewards and punishments can be set up, the staff must determine what each individual's desirable and undesirable behavior is. In general, desirable behavior leads to the goals the patient and staff members mutually establish at the patient's admission, and undesirable behavior contributes to the patient's fixation on pain.

For example, undesirable behavior for pain-clinic patients is talking about the pain at any time except when asked a specific question by the physician or other medical personnel. So if you start a conversation with a ward nurse about your pain, "My leg is really bothering me today; I don't think I'll get up and make my bed, and I also would like some more of that medication Dr. R. prescribed last week," the nurse will mete out "punishment"—she will ignore your statement.

Generally, if someone says something and is ignored, he will tend not to repeat the statement. Being ignored is embarrassing and frustrating, both unpleasant feelings. Most people like to avoid unpleasant feelings. As a result, when the nurse and others continually ignore your statements about your pain, you will avoid making them, and instead make statements that will lead to a conversational response. The punishment meted out reduces those forms of behavior that the staff wants you to avoid—your behavior has been modified.

On the other hand, if you exhibit a behavior on the ward that brings you closer to your goal, such as stretching your arm during a physical therapy session (when you have kept that arm immobile for many months), you will be verbally encouraged to continue that behavior. Encouragement is also accompanied by praise. For example, if you willingly follow the therapist's instructions and go a bit further than asked, she will praise you. Most people like praise—it acts as a reward. You will continue to try to win the praise (the reward) by doing just a little bit more for the therapist. By reinforcing what she has observed to be a good behavior in you, the therapist has helped you to modify your behavior. You no longer keep your arm immobile and you have moved a little farther on the path to your goal.

Most activities on the ward are fashioned to encourage modification of the chronic-pain patient's behavior. Making your bed, going to the nurses' station for your medication, or simply socializing by chatting with fellow patients are all behaviors that are encouraged. They are activities that will keep you functioning and lead you to a life outside your pain.

Behavior modification actually is a beginning to a new way of life. Its goal is to remove pain from your life as much as possible. If your behavior changes are successful, you reap all the rewards. You achieve other goals. Refocusing your thoughts and activities need not be the only end of behavior modification. You will relate to people differently if the method is successful. Relating to people differently, you will feel less depressed, better about yourself, and you will probably start believing that you can learn to tolerate your pain.

Motivation to achieve these goals is most clearly seen in this phase of treatment. The patient must have a sincere desire to be pain free or a sincere desire to resume a more normal life in order for behavior modification to truly work. The patient who is so motivated has a good chance for successful treatment.

The pain clinic, in some ways, can be compared to the therapeutic community concept. The therapeutic community is an alternative to placing drug abusers or alcoholics in jails or prisons. The whole purpose of the community, which is composed of a group of people with a common need and goal (to get off of drugs and remain drug free), is therapy. Every activity in the community is therapy. The therapy teaches the residents responsibility. They need to learn to be responsible for their own lives, as they forfeited that responsibility when they became addicted to drugs. Drug addiction is in part a life-style, so the therapeutic community shows the addict that there can be a different life-style that is fulfilling and useful.

With its behavior-modification program, the pain clinic also strives to teach the chronic-pain patient to take responsibility for his life and his health, rather than focusing on his disease. This should enable the patient to discard his former perceptions about the pain—of course, this all occurs in tandem with the other treatments that the pain clinic offers.

You can practice behavior modification on yourself without going to a pain clinic. For example, if you find yourself avoiding a party because the pain puts a damper on your spirits, make a special effort to go in spite of how you feel. You may have a good time and manage to forget the pain.

If you find you are doing less and less of what you want to do, get yourself a small notebook and write down what you have avoided doing when you feel the pain. Do this for several weeks.

Then look back at your notes and pick an activity that seems easy and work at doing it when you feel the pain again. Pick one activity at a time until you have tried them all again. You may have started coping with your chronic pain.

9
Drug Management
Relief Without Addiction

This chapter is about drug management: why certain drugs are selected to alleviate pain, how they work, and how physicians determine which ones to use for each patient. To aid in your understanding of this subject, we begin with the following list of the basic categories of drugs and their effects on your body. The categories are not rigid and in some cases a drug will fit into several of them.

Analgesics

Analgesics are drugs that relieve or allay pain. These drugs range from simple and ubiquitous aspirin to potent narcotics. Narcotics are substances that relieve pain as well as produce euphoria (a sense of well-being). Narcotics are habituating and can be addictive with long-term use.

Minor Tranquilizers

These tranquilizers are drugs that have a calming effect; they produce a peaceful feeling without inducing sleep. However, they can cause depression and rage reactions, and alter sleep patterns. They are usually addicting.

Major Tranquilizers

There are five major classes of drugs in this category. They are used to control psychotic behavior but can also be good antianxiety agents when taken in small doses. They are not addicting, but some can create shaking hands or lip tremor, which are usually controllable or reversible if detected early enough.

Hypnotics and Sedatives

These drugs produce a calming effect while they induce sleep. They usually are addicting and alter natural sleep. Barbiturates are among the most common sedatives, and they also act as hypnotics and are addicting.

Stimulants

Stimulants are any drug that increases or speeds up the functions and activities of the central nervous system. The amphetamines are the most common stimulants, and they also act as appetite suppressants for about two weeks. They are habituating and can cause depression with long use. Caffeine is a widely used stimulant.

Antidepressants or Mood Elevators

These are fairly new drugs, and they have the power to alter mood. Such drugs are prescribed to combat anxiety and fight off depression. They are not addicting or habituating, but some have uncomfortable side effects.

Hallucinogens

These drugs primarily produce hallucinations and as yet have not been found to have a medical purpose.

Muscle Relaxants

These are a specific group of drugs that reduce muscle spasms created by certain pain states. Some minor and major tranquilizers can also act as muscle relaxants.

Anti-inflammatory Agents

Beginning with aspirin and incorporating a host of steroids and steroidlike drugs, these agents reduce the swelling that can be associated with some chronic pain. The major side effect is stomach upset.

Vasoactive Compounds

These substances are designed to permit increased blood flow to damaged areas by increasing the diameter of blood vessels. Some of these drugs are useful for the treatment of headache.

In an effort to kill their pain, many patients spend years experimenting with a variety of therapies and physicians, and nothing works. During their long and fruitless search for a solution, many become addicted to drugs.

Addiction is a physical dependence on drugs; your body craves them and requires that you take them. The body becomes accustomed to drugs and needs them as it needs air and water. Because addiction causes chemical changes, the body will experience withdrawal symptoms without the substances on which it has come to depend. These symptoms can include shakes, sweats, cramps, and convulsions. Long-term use of addictive drugs can lead to altered personality, depression and, in some cases, can produce permanent residual brain damage.

Because of these undesirable side effects, narcotics, and the minor tranquilizers such as Valium and Librium, all of which have addictive potential, should not be considered the most beneficial analgesics on the market shelves. Yet they are the most frequently prescribed for chronic pain. What other drugs, then, can or should be used to reduce pain, anxiety, and depression? The answer to this question is directly related to what you have learned in previous chapters about the many factors that cause pain and affect one's perception of it.

Anxiety and Pain

One of the variables that must be taken into account when a physician prescribes a drug for acute pain is to what extent the patient's anxiety may be intensifying his pain. More than twenty-five years ago, one of the earliest pain researchers, Edward K. Beecher, M.D., studied acute pain and how it affected individuals in different locations and settings. He chose as his subjects a group of men who had been in combat and lay wounded on a battlefield. Because their injuries were so extensive, these soldiers had to be evacuated from the combat zone. The wounds varied in severity and involved different parts of the body, including chest and stomach wounds as well as multiple-fractured bones.

Dr. Beecher matched the soldiers' wounds to similar injuries sustained by a group of civilians who then needed to undergo major surgery in a hospital. The civilians also had chest and stomach wounds and compounded fractures.

Dr. Beecher found that the soldiers were less likely to request morphine than their civilian counterparts. He decided that the perception of acute pain, how much pain was felt or how much pain the patients were aware of, depended largely on how they perceived their immediate environment.

To the civilians, surgery meant disaster. Surgery meant being removed from comfortable and familiar objects at home and being placed in a frightening and sterile hospital. It meant coming face to face with the fact that they were ill, and this made the patients anxious. They were anxious about being ill and anxious about the outcome of the surgery.

For the soldiers surgery meant getting off the life-threatening battlefield to the relative comforts and safety of a hospital. It meant getting help for their wounds, and most of all, it meant getting out of war. The prospect of being evacuated to a field hospital for surgery was welcome. Therefore the soldiers did not experience the anxiety of their civilian counterparts, and according to Dr. Beecher, because of the reduced anxiety they perceived less pain. The evidence for this was that the soldiers made fewer requests for narcotics before surgery.

Dr. Beecher's theories about the effect of anxiety on the perception of pain were borne out by other researchers who found that a quantity of Thorazine, a potent tranquilizer used to calm violent mental patients, is equally as effective in reducing postoperative pain as a slightly smaller dose of morphine. Thorazine does not not have any of the analgesic power of morphine. Why then did the Thorazine work? It worked because of its calming effect.

According to many physicians, a great deal of postoperative pain is due to the patient's anxiety and general nervousness about the outcome of surgery. When patients enter surgery, they are anxious about the entire procedure. Some of the best surgeons are those who establish rapport with their patients, who talk to the patients prior to surgery, explaining at length what is going to happen to them, what techniques are going to be used, and what the patient should expect of himself after the surgery. Because knowing what to expect offers some measure of security, these patients are relatively calm going into the operating room and come out requesting less pain-killer.

Looking at the results these investigators achieved, it would seem that the physician should be able to avoid the use of narcotic analgesics—which are harmful when administered for long periods of time—if he can reduce his patient's anxiety, whether treating acute or chronic pain.

What drugs should be substituted for narcotics? Ideally, the chemical should fight anxiety, which eliminates some of the emotional components of pain, and have some pain reducing powers all of its own, without being addicting.

The phenothiazines are one such category of drug. Though they too have side effects, they are not nearly as severe in consequence as those of the benzodiazepines. For example, a physician might prescribe Valium as a tranquilizer hoping to reduce his patient's stress and anxiety about pain by calming him. However, the patient may become depressed, or may in fact have a paradoxical increase in his pain, due to the Valium (because of its chemical action), and the physician may eventually recommend that he see a psychiatrist because of these reactions. The psychiatrist may take the patient off Valium, and the patient may report either a lifting of depression, or a lessening of the pain. This phenomenon can be attributed to the action of Valium upon a drug in the brain called serotonin. Valium blocks the release of serotonin, which interferes with natural sleep, reduces the body's ability to tolerate pain, and, in some cases, may cause depression.

The phenothiazine tranquilizers are more effective against chronic pain, and have fewer potentials for depressive side effects. They are effective because they block receptor sites for two other chemicals in the brain (dopamine and norepinephrine) and the blocking of norepinephrine (nor-adrenalin) receptor sites increases pain tolerance. In doing this they also combat anxiety when administered in small doses. However, they too have side effects, such as restlessness and abnormal movements, and should be used with caution on a long-term basis.

Depression and Drugs

The use of antidepressant medication for chronic pain is a new, but promising, application of these drugs. There are basically three types of antidepressant medications available. These are the tricyclic antidepressants, monoamine oxidase inhibitors, and psychostimulants.

Depression is thought to be caused in some people by a chemical imbalance, specifically a deficiency of the neurotransmitters norepinephrine and serotonin. Therefore, it would appear that if these substances could be increased in the central nervous system, the depression could be alleviated.

It is now possible to biochemically differentiate two types of depression: first, a depression caused by a reduction of a drug in the brain called serotonin, and second, a depression caused by the reduction of the drug norepinephrine which, as noted above, is also in the brain. A reduction of either of these drugs may be accomplished by several means. Their receptor site activity can be artificially blocked by the administration of certain drugs, such as those used to treat high blood pressure. Or, the stores of these chemicals in the brain can be depleted by the use of other drugs, notably reserpine-containing compounds, which again are applied to the treatment of high blood pressure. Certain chemicals, such as Valium, can inhibit the release of serotonin, thereby causing depression, altered sleep patterns, and increased sensation of pain.

The *tricyclic antidepressants* reduce depression by increasing certain neurosynaptic transmitters (the chemicals in the brain of which we have recently talked—serotonin, norepinephrine, and dopamine). However, not all tricyclic antidepressants have the same effect, because they work on different neurosynaptic transmitters.

As discussed in Chapter 2, sensory nerves, such as pain fibers, are stimulated by the experience of a pain-producing sensation or event, such as extremes of temperature, pressure, and irritation. This stimulation is transmitted by a series of electrical impulses that travel along the nerve and cause the release of a chemical from the nerve ending. This chemical, which is called a neurosynaptic transmitter, or neurotransmitter (such as serotonin, norepinephrine, or dopamine), then takes over. The neurosynaptic transmitter jumps across a gap between two nerves (a synapse), binds to a specific receptor site on an adjacent nerve, and then chemically stimulates it to begin a series of electrical impulses along this second nerve. In less than a thousandth of a second this chemical is reabsorbed by the nerve that released it, and its action is thereby ended.

The important concept here is the specificity of these chemicals for one nerve or the other. As you can imagine, merely applying electrical current excites all types of nerves. However, by applying certain specific chemicals, one can excite or chemically block one type of nerve or another.

A moderate portion of this reabsorbed chemical is digested or used (metabolized) by the cell; it is broken down with the help of another chemical, or enzyme. This chemical is called monoamine oxidase.

All this brings us to *monoamine-oxidase inhibitors.* These chemicals work as antidepressants by increasing the concentration of available neurotransmitters—by inhibiting their metabolism by monoamine oxidase. If neurotransmitters are not metabolized, there will be more of them. If there are more of them, depression resulting from a deficiency of neurotransmitters can be relieved. Since the neurotransmitters serotonin and norepinephrine both are metabolized by monoamine oxidase, the monoamine-oxidase inhibitors allow the buildup of both chemical transmitters.

Psychostimulants function differently from the tricyclic and monoamine-oxidase-inhibitor-type antidepressants. They work by increasing the concentration of the desired neurotransmitter in the synapse by stimulating the release of the neurosynaptic transmitter from the pre-synaptic cell. In stimulating the release of the neurotransmitter, they generally stimulate the central nervous system. This is due to the release of a chemical called norepinephrine. This chemical in high concentration in the brain has been shown to increase the perception of pain. After a while, they can deplete the brain's supply of norepinephrine, and cause depression, or even a psychotic episode that looks like paranoid schizophrenia. Psychostimulants, therefore, are not the drug of first or even second choice to combat depression.

Rather than stimulate the chronic-pain patient's system, the physician wishes to sedate it to some degree, and the phenothiazine tranquilizers work well for this purpose. Within this group of tranquilizers are a subdivision, that are especially effective for chronic-pain patients, and have fewer sedative side effects than other drugs within this category. Drugs such as Stelazine, Prolixin, and Trilafon have less chance of producing drowsy, groggy side effects. Another drug that is not a phenothiazine, but in a completely different drug category, Haldol, has even fewer sedative side effects. However, the basic mechanism of action is the same. These drugs all work by blocking the post-synaptic reception of dopamine and norepinephrine. It has recently been shown that the blocking of norepinephrine lessens the perception of pain, and therefore produces some degree of relief.

Combinations of certain tricyclic antidepressants and some phenothiazines that do not have a sedative effect have been found useful for the treatment of pain from post-herpetic neuralgia and from intractable cancer. Research by Dr. Arthur Taub at Yale University has been confirmed by a variety of other investigators, which has led to the widespread use of the combination of Elavil and Prolixin.

Aspirin, of course, is one of the most common pain-killers in the world, and it is most effective for the treatment of pain from arthritis. Scientists as yet do not know exactly how it kills pain, but they suspect that it somehow activates the release of a substance called prostaglandin H, which acts as an analgesic at the pain nerve-fiber (free nerve endings). Unfortunately, too much aspirin can cause another type of pain—gastritis (stomach pain). This can be avoided by using a buffered compound that does not irritate the stomach lining as much as aspirin. (Scientists make breakthroughs in the arthritis field all the time and recently have announced some success with the use of lasers—powerful concentrations of pencil-thin light—in the fight against the pain of rheumatoid arthritis.)

Some chemicals when inhaled can cause severe facial pain. This pain can be combatted by anti-inflammatory drugs.

It is very difficult to relieve the pain of a patient who is dying from cancer or another disease that causes him to live in pain that can last for several years. Not too long ago, doctors were afraid to addict the dying patient who suffered a great deal of agonizing pain. They felt that to give them too much morphine, Demerol, Talwin, or Codeine would be wrong, because it could only lead to narcotic addiction. In recent years, however, attitudes about the dying have changed, and so has the attitude toward a more liberal use of narcotics for these patients.

In an attempt to avoid addiction some physicians experimented with the "P.R.N." concept. P.R.N. are the initials for the words per required need (administer as needed). In other words, the patient suffering from terminal bone cancer could not receive his medication until his last dose of narcotics had worn off and he was in pain again and needed the drug.

Much of the cancer patient's pain was probably due to the anxiety of anticipation: waiting to be hit with the pain again, hoping it wouldn't happen, tensing up because he knew it would. When physicians follow a fixed timetable for the administration of the drug, giving it to the patient every four hours, or preferably every three hours, since the effect of most narcotics lasts only 2½ to 3½ hours, the patient no longer anxiously awaits for the pain to hit again—because it won't. It will be stopped before the last dose of medication wears off. With his anxiety reduced, the patient's perception of pain also is reduced. In fact, doctors prescribing drugs on the fixed timetable find that their patients actually need less narcotics to maintain them in a pain-free state, rather than more, the "more" that leads to addiction.

American practitioners also have begun following in the footsteps of their counterparts in Britain, who for many years have given their terminal patients living in pain a "cocktail" whose ingredients include a narcotic, a stimulant, alcohol, and flavoring. This combination of drugs allows the patient to be pain free (the narcotic) while remaining alert (the stimulant), and the medication is made palatable by its flavoring.

Among the most promising drugs on the horizon are the body's own opiates, the endorphines and enkephalines (mentioned in Chapter 2). If the physician can learn to stimulate the natural opiates into action, he will be able to alleviate pain without the use of harmful drugs. The key to stimulating these drugs, however, is not known, but there are suggestions that the use of electrical stimulation, or acupuncture-like techniques may excite their production. Some of the most outstanding research in the field is conducted in the laboratory of Dr. Solomon Snyder, at Johns Hopkins University School of Medicine. Dr. Snyder, in conjunction with co-workers such as Dr. Gavril Pasternak (soon to become affiliated with the Memorial Sloan-Kettering Institute in New York City) and Dr. Mike Kuhar, as well as Dr. Candice Pert, formerly in Dr. Snyder's laboratory but now at the National

Institute of Mental Health outside Washington, D.C., is beginning research on the possibility of exciting the production of enkephalins, or finding the appropriate enzyme to create betaendorphin, from "big ACTH." (Big ACTH is a hormone, larger than regular ACTH, that is found in the pituitary gland. The initials stand for adreno-corticothrophic-hormone, which merely means a hormone that excites the outside layer of the adrenal gland.) If he is successful, he will have the gratitude of both patients and physicians alike.

The following is a list of the commonly prescribed drugs for chronic pain and an explanation of their basic action. (The list of brand names does not imply endorsement.)

Analgesics

Aspirin, buffered aspirin, and aspirin compounds are all over-the-counter drugs that are effective in combating headaches, muscular aches and pains, arthritis, sinusitis, and the aches and pains due to fatigue from overexertion. The buffered compounds contain an antacid to protect the stomach lining from the effects of aspirin. Many of the products contain caffeine, which acts as a diuretic and a general brain stimulant.

ASPIRIN PRODUCTS

Alka-Seltzer Effervescent Pain Reliever®
Alka-Seltzer Plus Cold Medicine®
Arthritis Strength Bufferin®
Ascriptin®
Bayer Aspirin®
Bayer Children's Aspirin®
Bayer Children's Cold Tablets®
Bufferin®
Congesprin®
Cope®
Coricidin®
Empirin Compound®
Excedrin®
Excedrin P.M.®
Vanquish®

NARCOTICS

Narcotics, some of which are derivatives of opium, are the most potent pain killers, and they are addictive.

The following narcotics are administered along with aspirin or aspirin-type compounds for the relief of all pain in all degrees of severity. If they prove ineffective the only stronger drug is morphine.

Ascriptin with Codeine®
Demerol Hydrochloride®
Dilaudid Hydrochloride®
Empirin Compound with Codeine Phosphate®
Emprazil-C Tablets®
Pavadon Elixir®
Percodan®
Sublimaze®
Tylenol with Codeine Tablets®

These narcotics are synthetics in combination with other chemicals.

Darvon®
Levoprome®
Talwin Compound®

The following are local anesthetics, used to produce a temporary state of numbing. These are the kinds of substances used in blocks.

Marcaine®
Novacain®
Xylocaine Hydrochloride®

Anti-inflammatory Agents

These drugs help fight pain by reducing swelling. The swelling may be caused by a variety of diseases, including gout, arthritis, and muscle damage.

Benemid®
Colchicine®
Indocin®
Motrin®
Napersin®
Telectin®
Zyloprim®

Antidepressants (or Mood Elevators)

These drugs work by reducing depression, and in some cases relieving anxiety. As mentioned in the chapter, they also work directly on the mechanisms of chronic pain.

Drugs working primarily on serotinin augmentation:
Anafranil® (not available in this country)
Adapin®
Elavil®
Sinequan®
Drugs that work both on serotonin and norepinephrine:
Imipramine Hydrochloride Tablets®
Tofranil Ampuls®
SK-Pramine Tablets®
Drugs that work primarily on norepinephrine:
Aventyl®
Desipramine®
Norpramine®
Vivactil®

Hypnotics and Sedatives

In low dosages, these drugs provide a calming effect, usually associated with drowsy side effects, while at higher dosages, these drugs induce a non-natural sleep. Most of the drugs listed below are addictive, interfere with the normal pattern of sleep, suppress the ability to dream, and may cause withdrawal symptoms upon the cessation of their use.

Aquachloral Supprettes®
Dalmane®
Luminal®
Placidyl®
Quaālude®

BARBITURATES

Alurate®
Amytal®
Butisol Sodium Elixir, Tablets®
Dialog®
Eskabarb Spansule Capsules®
Luminal®
Mebaral®

Nembutal Elixir®
Repan®
Seconal Elixir®
Tuinal®

NONBARBITURATES
Dalmane®
Equanil®
Miltown®
Placidyl®
Quāālude®
Sopor®
Tranxene®

Minor Tranquilizers, or Benzodiazepines

These drugs have a sedative and hypnotic effect. Some of these drugs also act to alter moods, may be addicting, and can cause depression. They have little or no use in the treatment of chronic pain.

Azine®
Librax®
Librium Capsules®
Serax®
Valium®
Tranxene®

Major Tranquilizers, or Phenothiazines and their Combinations

These drugs are not without their side effects, but they do inhibit the neurosynaptic transmitters, and can be useful in combating anxiety. They include Phenothiazines, Buterophenones, Phioxanthines, Molindones, and Dibenzoxazepines.

PHENOTHIAZINES
Compazine®
Mellaril®
Prolixin®
Serentil®
Stelazine®
Thorazine®

Trilafon®
Vesprin®

MAJOR TRANQUILIZERS WITH PHENOTHIAZINE-LIKE ACTION (BUTEROPHENONES, PHIOXANTHINES, MOLINDONES, DIBENZOXAZEPINES)

Haldol®
Loxitane®
Moban®
Navane®

Stimulants

These drugs increase the action of the central nervous system. They often are prescribed to counter the effects of sedative actions of analgesics.

AMPHETAMINES

Benzedrine Sulfate®
Biphetamine®
Desoxyn®
Dexamyl®
Dexedrine®
Didrex®
Eskatrol®

NONAMPHETAMINES

Sanorex®
Tenuate®
Tepanil®

Muscle Relaxants

These drugs reduce muscle spasms created by certain pain states.

Flexeril®
Robaxin®
Soma®
Valium Tablets® (a benzodiazepine, which may worsen pain)
Parafon Forte®

Vasoactive Compounds

These drugs permit more blood to flow to damaged areas by increasing the diameter of blood vessels. They can be useful in treating headache pain.

Cyclospasmol®
Gynergin®
Inderal®
Nicobid®
Octin®
Regitine®

10
Pain and the Family

As chronic pain takes center stage in the life of its victims, so too the chronic-pain patient becomes the focus of his family; he demands attention. His complaints disturb everyone in the household. His schedule of pills or doctor's examinations burdens the schedules of others and probably breaks the family's budget. Resentment builds. If family members do not cater to him, or if they try to ignore his constant indisposition and protestations of imminent collapse, the patient resents the "unfair" way he feels he is being treated. The family members, in turn, resent the amount of time the patient demands; they can understand that he doesn't feel well, but eventually they come to believe that the patient could feel better, could contribute more to the household if he truly wanted to. Chronic pain has the potential to destroy its victim's family as well as its victim.

Karen is a bright young woman who has always thought of herself as independent. As soon as she finished high school she said good-by to her family and set off on a cross-country tour of Europe on her own, hitchhiking all the way, against family advice. When she returned to this country, she decided to see it the same way and took another year before she settled down in a small apartment in her hometown. She decided to go to junior college, and her father offered to pay her tuition.

As soon as she finished school, she went into business for herself. She designed and produced greeting cards. She enjoyed what she was doing so much that she decided to do everything for herself, so she also started selling the cards, replacing her brother who had helped her with this part of the business. Both aspects of the work appealed to her—the artistic end appealed to her creative nature; selling her cards gave her an outlet for her aggressiveness.

Though Karen considered herself a loner, she accepted a marriage proposal from a department-store executive who had proposed not too long after she had sold him a batch of her greeting cards. Joe was an old-fashioned sort who insisted that his wife not work and that she settle down and raise all the children they planned to have. Karen fought him on this up until the day their first child was born, and then they reached a compromise. Karen would move her business into the house and simultaneously be a businesswoman and a full-time mother, as Joe felt she should be.

After two more children in as many years, Karen could not find much time for her business, and it started to fail. Just about the time Karen's business started doing poorly, she began to wake up in the morning with a low-back pain. Karen and Joe decided that their semisoft mattress was the culprit behind the pain and decided to buy a firmer one, but the harder mattress did not help her backache.

For the next few years, while she traveled from doctor to doctor looking for relief for her back pain, Karen was also trying to salvage her business. Eventually she was spending little time at home and moved her business back to an office building in the city. The move was accomplished only after some vicious arguments between her and Joe and a promise from Karen that all her free time would be spent with the children.

In addition to her emotional clashes with Joe over her business, the back pain kept on giving her trouble. It began to interfere with her sex life to the point where she told Joe that it was better for her if they had no sex at all, because the pain was too much to bear. Karen always seemed pressed for time. She felt tremendously guilty about neglecting her children while trying to reestablish her business—and felt angry about feeling guilty. She was also fatigued from the pain that did not allow her to get a good night's sleep. Karen's pain was fighting Joe and the three children for her attention—and winning.

But what about Joe and the three children: Where did they fit into Karen's life, particularly Karen's life marred by chronic pain?

By the time a psychiatrist referred Karen to a pain-treatment center, Joe was ready to leave her. He had often thought about disappearing one day and making a new life for himself in another state under a different name.

Joe was fed up with Karen and her pain. All he ever heard when he was home was that Karen didn't feel well and wanted to be left alone. He argued with her all the time. He felt that she was a rotten mother and a worse wife. He felt that during the past few years (since she had rekindled her business) she had become enormously self-centered and was ignoring everybody.

During the heat of one of their arguments, he finally told her that he didn't believe that she was really in pain. He told her that he felt that it was just an excuse to stay away from him. Karen admitted that she thought he had been running around with other women—he had before when she was pregnant—so she didn't see what difference it made to him that they were no longer having sex. Joe exploded when she said that and nearly hit her, but instead he left the house for two weeks. He told himself he just didn't want to hear about her pain anymore.

When he returned home, Karen suggested that they both enter family therapy at the pain-treatment center. Joe agreed. After their first meeting, the therapist requested that Karen and Joe bring the children to the sessions. He felt that Karen's pain probably had affected them, and that their behavior, in turn, probably had an effect on Karen, and on her pain.

During therapy Joe admitted that he felt left out of Karen's life, ignored and abused. He said that he understood that Karen's back hurt her, but on another level and after two years, he just couldn't believe that she really was in pain anymore. Believing this made him angry and made him want "to get even" with Karen for deceiving him, by hurting her and making her angry. Joe said he felt as if he were being pulled apart by his emotions, and he thought that the best thing for him to do would be to leave Karen permanently. He said that he saw no alternative to leaving, that most of his sympathy for Karen had been eroded by their quarrels and her complaints about pain.

The children appeared to be as upset as Joe over their mother's pain and her behavior. The children were young (ages eight, nine, and ten), but articulate. They all said that they didn't understand their mother anymore. She was not the same person they knew and loved when they were younger. It seemed that she picked on them all the time, and that nothing ever pleased her. They felt inadequate and ashamed, because they would do anything to avoid her and stay out of her way. She was too unpredictable for them; she would burst out screaming for almost any incident, and for spilling a glass of milk, one of them might get a severe beating. So they just avoided her.

The ten-year-old felt the brunt of his mother's chronic pain. As the oldest he had more freedom to do something about his situation. After a particularly bad night of pain, Karen started picking on him from the moment he got up until he went to sleep that night. So he ran away. Karen, feeling incapacitated by her pain, just called the police and had him picked up. He was placed in a juvenile facility until Karen came to get him. The ten-year-old ran away several more times—whenever his mother beat him or was especially unpredictable.

Because the father stayed away from home a lot, he was not aware how serious things were for his son. The child spent more time in a state facility than he should have and this had an effect on him. He was unmanageable, unmannerly, and did poorly in school. He said he hated his mother, he did not know why she changed, and he would like to have the old one back; if not, he did not want to live with his parents anymore.

The younger children were also confused and angry. They also didn't like to be near their mother. She had become a malevolent stranger to them, and they preferred to spend time at the homes of their friends. Whenever Karen complained about pain and asked one of them to bring her her pills, the youngest would start sucking her thumb and the nine-year-old would hide.

During the therapy session, Karen admitted that she was mortified by her family's behavior and believed that they did not care about her any longer. She had decided that disciplining them was useless, although in the back of her mind, she knew that they needed some firm discipline (dispensed with love). But she was too fatigued by her pain to discipline, so she yelled and hoped for the best.

Karen's family was falling apart and her pain was responsible.

Her pain made her unpredictable, savagely changing her from a warm (but aggressive) personality into someone who was strange and irritable and highly volatile. She caused her husband to feel angry, guilty, and deprived. She confused and overwhelmed her children, and she virtually destroyed herself. Chronic pain was the major cause of the situation in Karen's family.

There is another side to the story of chronic pain and the family. Some families feed on the pain of one of its members. Some families enjoy having someone dependent, someone to cater to, to bring pills to, to feed, to tend to. Such treatment makes the family feel useful and needed. But by doing this the family is keeping the patient in pain by making the pain useful to the patient: his pain becomes a major topic of conversation, a focus of the household duty roster, and a way of getting constant attention.

Pain may be useful for the mother who does not want her children to leave the house (and leave her). Pain is useful to the child who does not want to leave the security of his home. Pain can be used to keep a straying husband or a straying wife at home.

Pain can make the whole family sick, which is why pain clinics often recommend that all family members receive treatment. In order to change the patient's attitude toward his pain, the family that contributes to the existence of that attitude also needs treatment. The family attitude must be changed.

11
Pain and the Physician

Chronic pain, you have seen, can work an awful transformation on an ordinarily happy, well-adjusted personality and change it into one that is unrecognizable, unhappy, and maybe unlovable. Rarely, however, does the person undergoing this process realize that he is affecting his physician, who has watched him change and has had an almost equal stake in his recovery.

The average physician wants to take care of people and cure them—he's not just a prescription writer, a knee tapper, or someone who refers you to a consultant. He sees himself primarily as a healer, and he is concerned about his patients. Try to imagine, then, what it must be like for him when a patient who has trusted him with his most prized possession—his health—comes back to him time after time with the same complaint, still trusting and hoping that the physician can make him better.

When a patient does not respond after repeated attempts by the physician to cure him, the ordinary doctor goes through some changes, too. The physician who is confident about his skills and capabilities, secure in his knowledge that today's medical technology can help or cure almost any ailment, begins to feel inadequate, inept, and unskilled when a chronic-pain patient returns again and again, confronting him with his failure. The physician places a lot of the blame for this failure on himself. After all, he put in many years training to be a healer and has been practicing his art for a long time—why can't he help this patient?

Too often, physicians forget that medicine is an art and not yet an exact science. They forget or do not realize that chronic pain is a subjective experience that they cannot measure, that they cannot force into quantities or qualities that can be touched, deciphered, rearranged, or altered.

Many physicians are unaware of the myriad obscure and hard-to-diagnose diseases that cause chronic pain. So, although the physician wants to help his patient, he is confronted with his own inadequacies and is frustrated in his attempts. This frustration can turn into anxiety for him. After all, he has used all his skills and called upon all the tests known to science (and known to him) to diagnose what seems to be an obvious condition.

After some months the physician eventually asks himself whether the patient's condition could be something that doesn't exist at all. In order to maintain his own confidence and allay his own fears, he comes to the conclusion that the chronic pain is not organic. Since all the tests are negative, since he is unable to relieve it, the chronic pain must be psychosomatic. (Not all physicians come to this conclusion; some stick with the patient for years trying to whip the pain into submission.) In making this diagnosis the physician shifts the responsibility for the patient's condition *from* himself and *onto* the patient. The doctor has decided that if he can't see the pain, if his tests can't measure it, then it simply cannot exist, even if it must be forced out of existence by fiat.

This is not an indictment of those physicians. Most physicians do want to help. What this general conclusion indicates is that chronic pain is a complex, time consuming, elusive disease that can outwit anyone. Chronic pain provokes unpleasant feelings in its victims, and the attending physician eventually becomes a victim too.

The following case focuses on a physician attempting to respond to the problems and crises of a patient afflicted with chronic pain.

George is a forty-year-old auto mechanic who was injured in a car accident. George did not know that he was injured in any way until two to three days after the accident when he started to feel a sharp pain in the back of his neck that seemed to radiate outward, down his shoulder and right arm.

When the pain started, George went to his family doctor, Morris Smith, whom he had regularly visited for the past twenty years. Morris was a family friend who often went out to dinner with George and his wife on weekends.

Morris was concerned about George and ordered every test he could think of, including an electromyogram, a nerve velocity test, and several other very sophisticated neurological examinations. All through the testing procedures George tried not to move his arm and shoulder and complained of pain in those areas.

When the test results came back, they were negative. Morris called George back to his office and told him the results. George told him that the pain had gotten worse. George said that it seemed that the pain was worse when he tried to use his arm, and that it felt slightly better when he rested his arm on something soft, like a pillow. George confided in Morris that the pain presented something of a problem for him at work because he had to use both hands to be any good at most minor jobs.

Morris talked with George at length and probed for more information. He found out that the damp weather they had had the past month also seemed to make George's arm feel worse, but that an application of a heating pad followed by a rubdown (performed by George's wife) made his arm feel a little bit better.

Morris was worried. George was an old friend who trusted him to see him through medical problems, and so far he wasn't able to do anything more for George other than tell him to keep on doing the same things that gave him relief. Morris prescribed a pain-killer and a sedative and told George to come back to see him in a month if the pain did not get any better.

When George came back the next month, Morris was embarrassed. George complained that the heating pad barely worked anymore and the pain was so incapacitating that he was on the verge of leaving his job.

So Morris recommended that George go to see the best orthopedic surgeon in town. Morris called the surgeon in advance of the appointment to give him George's medical records and he requested that the surgeon please keep him informed as he was very concerned about his patient.

The orthopedic surgeon ran all the tests available and could find nothing out of the ordinary, so he bounced George back to Morris. Morris was getting angry with himself for not being able to help his patient, particularly a patient who was a friend, a friend in pain. Morris thought the pain might even be affecting the friendship.

Morris then suggested that George see a neurosurgeon. George said the he would go if Morris was certain that should be the next step. But he also told Morris that his insurance was running out, he couldn't keep up with the pace at work anymore, and he was going to have to quit. He was thinking of applying for Social Security disability payments, but his wife was reluctant. She couldn't face her friends if she felt that they knew she and her husband were on "welfare." Morris was upset when he heard that. He was also feeling helpless because all he could do was to recommend this second consultation—it resulted in the neurosurgeon sending George on to a neurologist who also found nothing.

Meanwhile, the Social Security board, in reviewing George's application, sent George back to three more doctors: an orthopedic surgeon, a neurologist, and a neurosurgeon. Though they were different people from the first three specialists he had consulted, they all told him the same thing.

During all his visits to physicians, George from time to time called Morris to tell him about the latest reviews his pain received. Morris was already aware of all the consultation results, as the physicians had all called him to obtain George's medical records.

By now Morris was beginning to feel suspicious. He began to think that if seven physicians could find nothing wrong with George, perhaps, in fact, nothing was wrong.

Morris decided that George probably was faking the pain in order to get the disability payments and therefore have an excuse to retire. He just could no longer believe that something was wrong. He had done his best, and now he felt that George, perhaps, was using him, or that possibly the pain was all in George's head. He preferred to think that rather than to think that his friend was using him.

Finally, Morris referred George to an anesthesiologist who specialized in nerve blocks. After performing several tests, the anesthesiologist told him that he was not a suitable candidate for a nerve block.

George ended his odyssey in Morris' office. But Morris was no longer prepared to deal with his pain. George represented a mystery to him, as well as a failure. Since he could not cure him, perhaps, he thought, a psychiatrist could; and that is what he told George, though not exactly in those words. George was angry and left Morris's office feeling resentful, but he went to see the psychiatrist.

After evaluating George's psychological history, the psychiatrist decided that he was not a malingerer. He ordered a thermography test and found that there was an area of pain in his shoulders. He decided to test George for myofascial syndrome by pressing on two trigger points in the area that he complained about. George yelped in pain. The psychiatrist explained that feeling the pain at the trigger points indicated that he probably was a victim of primary myofascial syndrome. George was relieved to know that his pain was "real" after all, even though so many doctors had implied that the pain did not really exist.

What about Morris; how did he feel? By the time Morris sent George to the psychiatrist, he was feeling inept, inadequate, embarrassed, and confused. If George ever returned to his office, Morris knew their relationship could never be the same. George represented failure to him. George probably never knew how desperately Morris wanted to cure him and probably will not return to Morris. Morris, it seems, loses on all counts.

Most physicians are similar to Morris in that they try to do their best to heal or cure their patients, they see failure to heal or cure as a personal and professional disaster. (There is, however, one kind of chronic-pain patient who is offensive to the physician. This is the malingerer, as described in Chapter 5. The malingerer, who consciously tries to deceive the doctor for his own personal gain, can make the most patient physician lose control and objectivity.) Chronic-pain patients always represent a challenge, but they also are symbols of potential failure and for this reason may frighten some physicians.

Appendices

What Price Relief?

The Cost of Treatment at Pain Clinics

Some sociologists and economists and others who have written on the subject have speculated that many chronic-pain patients may spend as much as $25,000, in some cases more, in their search for relief.

This vast amount of money pays for physicians' fees, the endless amount of drugs consumed, surgery and hospital bed space, psychiatric bills, and travel. This dollar figure, of course, does not take into account how much is spent in time and personal energy looking for relief, nor does it consider the cost borne by the patient's family.

How much will you spend in a pain clinic? We cannot give you a definitive answer as costs vary from city to city, coast to coast, and are subject to change with the vagaries of the inflation rate. The cost depends not only on geographic location but also on the orientation of the clinic (the cost will be more in a clinic where there is an emphasis on tests and diagnostic evaluation than in a less academically inclined facility).

To give you some idea of the range of cost, one pain clinic, a medical school hospital on the eastern seaboard, charges between $5,000 to $10,000 for a three-week stay. This does not cover the cost of prescribed items such as medications or electrical stimulators, which can run between $100 and $300. The total cost per week averages $3,000. However, a private clinic nearby, using medical school affiliated physicians, costs $1,500 a week. At a southern pain-treatment center affiliated with a hospital, for a pain patient routinely admitted for a two-week stay, the basic room rate is about $100 a day, and then the patient has to pay each individual specialist his set fee, which can run $200 to $300. Total costs can run $2,500 a week. Another southern hospital charges a flat $1,500 a week for treatment. This amount does not include the cost of your motel while you receive the initial three-day evaluation on an out-patient basis, increasing the total costs for the week to $2,000. Another clinic might charge $500 for an evaluation and suggested treatment.

All these expenses do not necessarily have to come out of your pocket. Your insurance plan can pick up some, if not most, of the costs, depending on the type of services you receive. You have to examine your insurance policy to determine whether or not you can be reimbursed for services and physicians' fees. It's important to remember that while recommended prescription items may not be paid for, your prescription bill is likely to be reduced rather than increased when you are finished with your treatment at the pain clinic. Talk to the insurance company to find out what they will pay for; it never hurts to ask, and you may be surprised at how much is covered. Also, it may be useful to discuss financial arrangements with the pain clinic staff. These people often have experience with the many different insurance carriers, and they may be able to help you decipher exactly what benefits are due to you.

If you are eligible, Medicaid and Medicare will pick up some of the costs of a pain-treatment center. Medicare will pay for some clinical services and some of the electrical stimulator devices. Medicaid payment varies, according to what each state's plan picks up as optional services. Again, inquire from the local board before checking into the clinic.

Regardless of the cost of the chronic-pain-treatment center, we can only offer the following advice. Seek out chronic-pain-treatment facilities that have academic affiliations. Additionally, find a center that uses a multidisciplinary approach to the diagnosis and treatment of chronic pain, and be wary of any pain clinic that makes exaggerated claims for success. Avoid any clinic that uses a single modality of treatment for all types of pain, and that fails to provide any diagnostic evaluation prior to beginning treatment. Check the credentials of the physicians who are associated with the chronic-pain-treatment center—this may be done through the *Marquis Compendium of Medical Specialists.* If a physician is listed in this reference text, this means he has been certified by the medical board in his specialty, and has exhibited a degree of competence within a given field. This does not imply that physicians who are not board certified are not qualified, nor that those who are certified are qualified, but certainly it does provide some guideline when seeking medical attention. Avoid any chronic-pain-treatment center that advocates the use of narcotics, analgesics, hypnotics, or sedative drugs. There is no pharmacological rationale for the use of these drugs in the treatment of chronic pain, unless it is intractable cancer pain. The physician who subscribes to this therapy is not as well-informed as he may be about the treatment of chronic pain.

A List of Pain Clinics

The following is a list of pain clinics in the United States. These are by no means all the pain clinics, but do represent most of the multidisciplinary pain-treatment centers. In order to locate the clinic nearest to you, you can write to your local medical society or to the American Association of Anesthesiologists in Arlington Heights, Illinois.

Baptist Hospital
Miami, Florida 33101

City of Hope Medical Center
Los Angeles, California 90052

Johns Hopkins University School of Medicine
Pain Treatment Center
Baltimore, Maryland 21205

Mensana Clinic
Stevenson, Maryland 21153

Mount Sinai Hospital
Pain Consultation Center
Miami, Florida 33101

New York University Medical Center
School of Medicine
New York, New York 10016

Rush Presbyterian-St. Luke's
Medical Center Pain Clinic
Chicago, Illinois 60607

Scripps Clinic
Pain Treatment Center
Claremont, California 91711

University of Illinois
School of Medicine
Pain Clinic
Chicago, Illinois 60612

University of Miami
School of Medicine
Pain Evaluation Team
Miami, Florida 33101

University of Washington
School of Medicine
Pain Clinic
Seattle, Washington 98195

Pain Unit
Lourdes Hospital
Binghamton, New York 13902

Cox Pain Center
San Luis Obispo, California 93401

Boston Pain Unit
Massachusetts General Hospital
Boston, Massachusetts 02114

Medical Center
Del Oro Hospital
Houston, Texas 77002

University of Virginia
Medical Center
Pain Clinic
Richmond, Virginia 23219

Emory University
Emory Clinic
Pain Control Center
Atlanta, Georgia 30333

University of Pittsburgh
Pain Control Center
Pittsburgh, Pennsylvania 15261

University of California-Los Angeles
Pain Control Unit
Los Angeles, California 90024

Glossary

acetominophen (Tylenol): a chemical that can reduce pain and fever, but does not have the antiinflammatory properties of aspirin.

acetylcholine: one of the neurosynaptic transmitters. This chemical is located in the brain and the parasympathetic system. Like norepinephrine (see below) it has specific receptors in blood vessels, nerves, and muscles. The action of acetylcholine usually is antagonistic to the action of norepinephrine.

acupuncture: the insertion of needles in and around the nerve, producing numbness in the surrounding area. The effects usually are not long lasting and require repeated application.

adiction: a physiological state in which a person develops a tolerance to a particular drug and needs ever increasing dosages of the drug to obtain the same effect. Also, when the drug is no longer taken, the person experiences "withdrawal" symptoms, which indicate the existence of a physical dependence on this chemical. This reaction is found with opiates, barbiturates, and benzodiazapines.

adhesion: a band of fiberlike material on the surface of a membrane that connects to the surface of another membrane, as an adhesion between one side of a wound and another.

analgesia: a loss of the sensation of pain.

analgesic: any compound that relieves pain without producing anesthesia or loss of consciousness.

anesthesia: generally a state characterized by a loss of any sensation caused by the depression of nerve function either with drugs or by disease.

anesthesiologist: a physician who specializes in the

administration of chemicals that produce a sleeplike state with some reduction of pain sensation for patients prior to operations. Also, these physicians are skilled and trained in injecting various areas of the body to produce pain relief.

antidepressant: any chemical that relieves the feeling of depression.

antihistamine: the body contains histamine, which causes a variety of symptoms, such as runny nose, red eyes, and excessive mucous formation. Any medication that blocks the action of histamine is called an antihistamine.

anxiety: a dread or fear of danger that can be accompanied by tension, restlessness, or palpitations; usually there is no clearly identifiable reason for these feelings of apprehension.

arthritis: a medical disease that may be caused by a local inflammation in a joint, damage to the joint itself, or by some infection. There are a number of different forms of this disease, variously called rheumatoid, osteo, and gonorrheal arthritis. Any inflammation of a joint, regardless of the ideology, is an arthritis.

atrophy: a reduction in size of a muscle group due to lack of use, which may occur either on a voluntary or involuntary basis (see paralysis).

axon: the part of the cell that conducts nervous impulses to dendrites away from the body cell. The axon looks somewhat like a filament and varies in thickness and length, up to fifty centimeters long.

axonal: pertaining to a nerve axon. A nerve axon is the long, pipelike tube that connects the cell body at one end to the terminal ending that contains neurosynaptic transmitters.

Briquet's syndrome: people with Briquet's syndrome usually have a variety of minor physical complaints, but because they generally have had moderate to severe psychiatric difficulties beforehand, they are overwhelmed by these difficulties and dwell on them.

bursitis: an inflammation of the sac covering a joint (the sac contains a fluid that lubricates the joint). When this covering is inflamed, it produces a syndrome that may be mistaken for arthritis, but is in actuality bursitis. It is usually accompanied by swelling and increased fluid in the area around the joint.

causalgia: a severe persistent burning sensation in the skin normally following an injury, either direct or indirect, to the sensory fibers of a peripheral nerve.

classical conditioning: in this technique, described by Pavlov, an animal or human is trained to respond to a stimulus to which he normally would not react. He eventually begins to respond to what previously had been a neutral stimulus with almost the same degree of intensity as he responds to a natural stimulus. The standard example of this process was Pavlov's pairing of the sound of a bell with the presentation of food in order to get a dog to salivate. In time, the sound of the bell alone was enough to induce salivation.

barbiturate: a drug that is a central nervous system depressant; it slows down the activities of the central nervous system.

behavior modification: this is a psychological technique by which a form of behavior is altered, without regard to the motivation that has produced it. In this technique, analogous to training a dog or a cat, a series of psychologicial maneuvers, such as the dispensing of rewards and punishment and the shaping of behavior, are used.

benzodiazepines: these are a group of chemicals that are the "minor tranquilizers" and are the most prescribed drugs in the United States today. These produce anxiety reduction, but may create addiction, dependence, and a variety of other undesirable side effects, including depression.

biofeedback: this is a newly developed technique by which certain body functions, such as temperature and muscle tension, which a person cannot measure by himself, are measured for him by an instrument and "fed back" to him. By virtue of this ability to visualize bodily functions, a person can then gain control over functions that he previously could not control.

block: arresting the passage of a nervous impulse usually by injecting a chemical, either alcohol or a local anesthetic solution, directly into the nerve.

dementia: this is the loss of memory and ability to reason that may be caused by a variety of problems, such as old age, with concomitant blockage of blood vessels to the brain. In this case, it is called senile dementia. Alcohol, other chemical substances, vitamin deficiencies, and some neurological diseases may causes other types of dementia.

dendrite: a branch of a nerve cell that receives nerve impulses from the axon of a neighboring nerve.

denervation: an operation that cuts off the nerve supply to a particular part of the body by incision, excision, blocking, or burning the nerve.

depression: a dejected feeling where the person feels so bad or low that it is readily discernible to others. Depressions are either reactive (in response to a situation such as the loss of a loved one) or endogenous (coming from within and having no discernible external cause such as the loss mentioned above).

dopamine: a neurosynaptic transmitter usually found in the brain that is specifically associated with some forms of psychosis and abnormal-movement disorders. This chemical also causes vessels to constrict.

dystrophy: literally means defective nutrition. Sympathetic reflex dystrophy refers to a painful illness that has a spreading or burning sensation, usually occurs in a limb, and leads to a restriction in motion in the affected limb. Trauma is a major cause of sympathetic reflex dystrophy.

electrical stimulators: see transcutaneous stimulators.

electromyographic: this refers to the measurement of the electrical component of muscle action. Every time a nerve sends information to the muscle to make it move, an electrical impulse travels down the nerve, causing the release of a chemical. The electrical impulse can be measured by a variety of instruments such as EMG (electromyographic) biofeedback instruments, and EMG (electromyogram) machines.

endorphin: a naturally produced chemical that has a morphinelike action and is usually found in the brain. High concentrations of endorphin are believed to cause the relief of pain and may be the body's own protection against pain.

enkephalin: like endorphin, a naturally produced chemical that has a morphinelike action. Enkephalin is usually found in the brain and the spinal cord, and its action is analogous to endorphin's.

etiology: the cause of a disease.

euphoria: a feeling or sensation of well-being. Sometimes an exaggerated feeling of being on top of the world physically as well as emotionally.

facet: a small smooth area on a bone, or a place that has been worn away on a smooth, firm structure.

facet blocks: this is a test done either by an anesthesiologist or a neurosurgeon, in which a numbing substance (local anesthetic) is injected in and around a nerve found on the bony surface of the vertebrae in the back. In some instances this injection can reduce or eliminate some painful syndromes of the back.

fascia: covering over the muscle that allows it to glide over adjacent muscle.

gate theory: an attempt to explain the mechanism by which the sensation of pain is reduced through the intentional irritation of areas in the same nerve distribution as the sensation. Basically, it says that if you overload a pathway, it will not be able to transmit all the messages it receives and will selectively decide to eliminate the painful transmission.

generic: the non-trademark name for a drug; its class.

housemaid's knee: a form of bursitis (see above) that is caused by repeated injury (such as constant kneeling) to the covering of the knee joint.

hypnosis: a repetitive series of statements that alters the attention of its subject and makes him extremely receptive to suggestions.

hypnotic: any chemical that, after administration, allows the person to sleep.

hysterical conversion: this is an unconscious defense against a horrible psychological trauma. In most cases the patient is overwhelmed or overcome by something they have thought, seen, or experienced. In order to cope with this trauma, the patient develops a symptom, such as blindness, paralysis, or spasm, which then can account for the severity of his reaction.

iatrogenic: resulting from the administrations or activities of a physician or surgeon.

innervation: the actual supply of nerve fibers to a particular part of the body.

ischemia: a reduced blood flow to part of the body.

keloid: an overgrowth of scar tissue that far exceeds the normal growth of scar tissue for a given injury.

Lamaze method: a technique for assisting childbirth that consists of informing the mother of the various stages of delivery prior to the onset of labor and instructing both parents in a routine that has hypnoticlike qualities. The result is the reduction of the anxiety and pain associated with childbirth.

lesion: a wound or injury, or any change in tissue.

limbic system: an area in the brain associated with the control of emotion, eating, drinking, and sexual activity.

MMPI (Minnesota Multiphasic Personality Inventory): a 566-question test that asks true-false questions. The patient takes this test himself, and then a psychologist scores it and interprets personality characteristics.

monoamine oxidase: an enzyme found in the nerve endings that breaks down certain neurosynaptic transmitters, such as serotonin, norepinephrine, and dopamine. By blocking this chemical with the use of monoamine oxidase inhibitors, an accumulation of these neurosynaptic transmitters can occur.

monoamine oxidase inhibitors: a group of chemicals used to treat depression, in some instances phobic anxiety, and may have some limited application in the treatment of pain. (See above.)

multidisciplinary pain-treatment center: a pain-treatment center where the emphasis is placed on diagnosis of the origin of the painful syndrome. This involves the input of a variety of physicians, including neurosurgeons, neurologists, orthopedic surgeons, anesthesiologists, psychiatrists, psychologists, and, on occasion, rheumotoidologists, internists, and endocrinologists. After the diagnosis has been established, treatment is begun in a two-prong fashion: treatment of the physical causes and effects of pain and an effort to help the person deal with the psychological problems caused by the pain.

muscle guarding: when an area of the body is damaged, there is an involuntary response called muscle guarding that manifests itself as increased muscle tension over the injured area.

myelin: a proteinlike material that envelops the axons of nerve fibers. It is composed of alternating layers of fats (lipid) and proteins. Myelin is analogous to the insulation on an electrical wire, allowing electrical impulses to remain within the nerve bundle without spreading to adjacent nerves.

myofascial syndrome: *myo* means muscle and *fascial* means the covering over the muscle that is very smooth and allows one muscle group to glide freely across another muscle group. When the muscle is damaged by an injury to the body, blood and other substances get into the space between muscles that is separated by the fascial covering. A scar, or an adhesion, is then formed in this area and the muscles are prevented from gliding smoothly over one another. The result is muscle spasm, and later, pain.

narcotic: any substance producing a stuporlike state while it kills pain; more specifically, a drug derived from opium or opiumlike compounds that can affect mood and behavior and has a potential for dependence and tolerance.

nerve: a whitish cord made up of fibers arranged in bundles and held together with connective tissue (myelin).

neuralgia: nerve pain that feels like severe throbbing or stabbing along the nerve pathway.

neuritis: an inflammation of a nerve that may be caused by a viral infection, mechanical irritation, or reduced blood flow. This may manifest as a burning sensation, exquisite increase in sensitivity, paralysis, numbness, or muscular atrophy in areas of the body (skin and muscle) supplied by the nerve.

neuroleptic: any chemical that can serve as a tranquilizer with specific antipsychotic actions is called a neuroleptic. This is a category of drugs, rather than one specific drug.

neuroma: when a nerve is crushed as the result of an injury, a number of chemicals are released that help it to regenerate and restore its function. However, the injury usually destroys the channels through which the nerve should grow, so that sensory nerves, especially pain nerves, develop into a tangled, bird's nest pattern. This mass of tangle of free nerve endings is called a neuroma, and is exquisitely painful to the touch.

neuron: the nerve cell.

neurosis: a psychological or behavior disorder in which anxiety plays a prime part. People with neuroses do not necessarily exhibit a gross distortion of reality; more often they have phobias or are unable to cope with stress situations.

neurosynaptic transmitter: same as neurotransmitter.

neurotransmitter: a chemical released by the pre-synaptic cell that crosses the synapse to inhibit or excite the post-synaptic cell.

norepinephrine: one of the neurosynaptic transmitters, this chemical is found in the brain and in the endings of some sympathetic nerves. There are specific receptors for norepinephrine located in a variety of tissue such as the blood vessels, nerves, and specialized muscles like the heart. Sometimes the blocking of this chemical can reduce pain sensations.

normal: healthy according to a standard.

operant conditioning: this is a technique developed by Thorndike, and expanded by Skinner, by which animals and humans (see behavior modification above) can be trained to do certain tasks by using a system based on the meting out of rewards and punishment and the shaping of behavior. The important factor here is the use of a reward when a desired behavior is achieved.

organic: related to the body (as opposed to the mind), such as a disease that is organic in origin; that is, starting in or caused by some organ (any part of the body that has a specific function).

opiate: any chemical derived from opium that produces pain relief and a state of well-being.

palatal myoclonus: this very rare syndrome is caused by damage to specific motor centers in the brain stem (the lower portion of the brain). It is manifested as a spasmodic contraction in the soft palate, located at the upper-rear portion of the mouth.

paleospinothalamic tract: an area in the spinal cord that runs alongside the neospinothalamic tract and becomes active when painful stimulation is constant and chronic (lasting longer than six months). This tract reaches areas in the brain in addition to the thalamus, eventually involving areas of the hypothalamus and limbic system, thereby creating the emotional components associated with chronic pain.

paralysis: the loss of power or voluntary control over the use of a muscle due to injury or disease of its nerve supply. The damage may occur anywhere along the pathway from the brain, spinal cord, specific nerve, or the junction between the nerve and muscle. This may result in atrophy of the muscle due to disuse.

paranoia: a mental disorder marked by delusions that the person is being persecuted and that he is special. Often a paranoid personality has an otherwise normal grasp of reality.

percutaneous rhizotomy: the permanent destruction of a nerve coming from the spinal cord that carries the sensory fibers from a particular area of skin and muscle. The procedure involves the insertion of a needle through the skin and muscle to the nerve to be destroyed, using an X-raylike device (fluoroscope) for direct visualization and the application of electrical current to burn away the sensory component of the nerve.

phantom limb pain: when an appendage, such as an arm or leg, has been traumatically amputated, very often the person will continue to report a sensation of pain, itching, or burning in the missing limb. This indicates that the brain is still receiving messages from the severed nerve fibers and is interpreting them as if the limb were still present.

phenothiazines: a group of tranquilizers, or neuroeleptics, that are specifically used for the treatment of psychoses. At lower dosages they can be useful for the treatment of anxiety and, in some instances, for the treatment of pain states, since they interfere with the chemicals that transmit painful messages.

phlebogram: a test in which dye is injected into the venous system, and photographs (a series of X-rays) are taken in order to ascertain whether there is any obstruction in the veins.

placebo effect: anytime a substance or activity can produce a desired result without the use of what is considered an active agent, this is termed a placebo effect. This phenomenon is poorly understood, but basically indicates that a patient who receives attention, regardless of the type of medication or manipulation administered, will derive benefit from the personal contact.

pleurisy: just as the muscles have a covering called the fascia, the lungs have a covering known as the pleura. When this covering is inflamed, breathing becomes painful. Any inflammation of the pleura is called pleurisy.

post-herpetic neuralgia: any irritation or inflammation of a nerve that is the result of an infection that is caused by the herpes virus. The most common post-herpetic neuralgia is herpes zoster (shingles) and trigeminal neuralgia.

psychoanalysis: a method of psychotherapy originated by Sigmund Freud in the nineteenth century that attempts to bring unconscious or subconscious material to the patient's conscious, then analyze it for therapeutic benefit.

psychogenic: of mental origin; related to psychic processes of behavior, personality, and other psychological processes.

psychoses: a mental disorder affecting a person's organization of thoughts, perception of reality, ability to communicate with other people, and capacity to cope with daily stresses and demands. Psychoses may be caused by severe emotional stress, biochemical abnormalities in the brain, or the natural aging process, resulting in organic brain syndromes. Certain drugs also may induce psychoses.

psychostimulants: these are a group of chemicals that excite the entire brain. Caffeine and amphetaminelike substances may be included in this group.

receptor: a specialized area on a nerve membrane, a blood vessel, or a muscle, which receives the chemical stimulation that activates or inhibits the nerve, blood vessel, or muscle.

reflex sympathetic dystrophy: a disorder of the sympathetic nervous system, due to either entrapment or damage. The critical manifestations are tingling, pins and needles sensations, and coldness in the affected limb. In extreme forms, hair loss, and loss of bone from the fingertips or toetips is visible on X-rays. This disorder can easily be detected with the use of thermography.

schizophrenia: the most common type of psychosis, characterized by delusions, hallucinations, and a withdrawal from relationships with other people into a world of one's own. Schizophrenia is thought to be a group of disorders rather than a single illness.

SCL 90-R: this is a test very similar to the MMPI (see MMPI above), but it contains only 90 questions compared to the MMPI's 566. This test also has the capacity to measure changes in the person's response over time, which the MMPI does not.

sedative: any chemical that calms a person down: it also produces drowsiness.

sensation: the translation of a stimulus into a consciousness of the effects of the stimulus; a feeling.

serotonin: a chemical found in the brain and in some areas of the intestine, as well as in circulating blood. There are receptors for this chemical in the brain associated with the relief of depression, in the vessel walls associated with an intense constriction of the vessel, and in the intestines associated with increased bowel motility.

somatogenic: a disorder or disease with clear-cut physical origins. *Soma* means body and *genic* is a term for arising from.

spinothalamic tract: this is an area in the spinal cord that transmits pain messages from the skin and muscles to the area of the brain that receives painful inputs.

steroid: a class of chemicals sharing a common structure that almost always function as hormones. These hormones are produced by the glands, including the ovaries or testicles and the adrenal gland.

sympathetic nerve blocks: in several painful syndromes (reflex sympathetic dystrophy), a numbing injection in the area of the sympathetic nerves may produce relief. If this is done repeatedly permanent relief may sometimes be obtained from a variety of the painful syndromes.

synapse: the gap between the membrane of one nerve cell and the membrane of another. The synapse is the point at which the transmission of nerve impulses occurs.

syndrome: the combination of signs and symptoms of a morbid process that constitutes a disease.

temporomandibular joint: a joint located between the bones of the skull and the lower jaw. This is the most unusual joint in the human body—the only one that can move in three directions: side to side; forward and back in a gliding fashion; in a hingelike opening motion. Damage to this joint, either by excessive grinding of the teeth (bruxism), or by injury to the muscle attaching the jaw to the skull (myofascial syndrome) can create a painful syndrome called temporomandibular joint syndrome.

tennis elbow: this is the result of repeated injury to the ligaments and tendons that hold the elbow joints together. This may be tendonitis, or, in some cases, an arthritis. This is due to repeated injury to a joint by excessive use.

thalamus: an area in the brain that receives pain messages from the spinothalamic tract and sends these messages to the cortex, which allows the perception and realization of pain.

thermocoagulation: the technique employed for performing a percutaneous rhizotomy. This means the application of a high-temperature probe, usually produced by the passage of electrical current, which selectively burns away the smaller sensory or pain carrying nerves, leaving the larger, motor nerves intact.

thermography: a specialized test to detect temperature differences caused by cancer growth or by injuries to the nervous system or blood vessels. Using heat-sensitive detection devices, a photograph may be taken in which the damaged area shows up as either warmer (in the case of cancer) or colder (in the case of pain that is caused by damaged vessels) than the rest of the body.

tic douloureux: a painful and sometimes disabling syndrome accompanied by horribly sharp shooting pains in the face. This is a synonym for trigeminal neuralgia.

CT scan (or CAT or tomographic scan): this is a newly developed test that takes a multiple group of X-rays from a variety of angles, and provides a three-dimensional view of certain of the areas under investigation. This has replaced several painful and sometimes dangerous tests.

transcutaneous stimulators: these are devices that emit an electrical current, which takes away certain types of pain. They are small devices that can be worn continuously and are available from a variety of sources.

trauma: an injury caused by rough contact with a physical object; an accidental or inflicted wound.

tricyclic antidepressants: a group of chemicals that are used to treat depression and, in some instances, to treat chronic pain.

trigeminal neuralgia: an irritation of the fifth cranial nerve, one of the nerves in the face. This irritation is usually caused by either a mechanical abrasion of the nerve or by a viral infection. This is also called tic douloureux.

Bibliography

Adolphe, Allen B., Ph.D.; Dorsey, Richard E., M.D.; Napoliello, Michael J., M.D. "Neuropharmocology of Depression." *Diseases of the Nervous System.* 38(1977):841–46.

Axelrod, Julius. "Neurotransmitters." *Scientific American.* 230(1974):58–71.

Beecher, H. K. "Relationship of Significant Wounds to Pain." *Journal of the American Medical Association.* 161(1956):1607–13.

Breuer, Josef, and Freud, Sigmund. "On the Psychical Mechanisms of Hysterical Phenomena." *Preliminary Communication (1893) in Studies on Hysteria.* New York: Avon Books, 1966, pp. 37–52.

Brown, Burnell, Jr., M.D., Ph.D. "Diagnosis and Therapy of Common Myofascial Syndromes." *Journal of the American Medical Association.* 239(1978):2386–89.

Drugs of Abuse, 4th ed. Washington, D.C.: U.S. Dept. of Justice, Drug Enforcement Administration, 1977. Produced by the Office of Public Affairs in Cooperation with the Office of Science and Technology.

Eccles, Sir John. "The Synapse." *Scientific American.* 212(1965):52–66.

Freud, Sigmund. "Fixation upon Trauma: The Unconscious." *A General Introduction to Psychoanalysis.* New York: Washington Square Press, 1963, pp. 284–96.

Funt, Lawrence, D.D.S., M.S., and Stack, Brendon, D.D.S., M.S. "The Evolution of the Craniomandibular Pain Syndrome, F.S. Index." *Clinical Management of Head, Neck and T.M.J. Pain and Dysfunction.* Edited by Harold Gelb.

Philadelphia: W. B. Saunders Company, 1978.

Gehris, C. W., Jr., M.D.; Hendler, Nelson, M.D. "Myoclonus Presenting as a Pulsatile Neck Mass." A paper presented at the eighty-first annual meeting of the American Academy of Ophthalmology and Otolaryngology, 6–10 October 1976, at Las Vegas.

"The Great Imposter: Diseases of the Temporomandibular Joint." *Journal of the American Medical Association.* Commentary. 235(1976):2395.

Hancock, Elise. "To Sleep: Perchance to Dream." *Johns Hopkins Magazine.* 84(1977):29–35.

Hendler, Nelson H., M.D. "Group Therapy with Pain Patients." Chapter 15 in *Diagnosis and Non-Surgical Management of Chronic Pain.* New York: Raven Press, 1979.

———. "Psychiatric Considerations of Pain." Chapter 104 in *Textbook of Neurosurgery.* Edited by J. Youmans, M.D., Ph.D. Philadelphia: W. B. Saunders Company, 1979.

———. "Psychopharmacology of Chronic Pain." Chapter 14 in *Diagnosis and Non-Surgical Management of Chronic Pain.* New York: Raven Press, 1979.

Hendler, Nelson, M.D.; Derogatis, Leonard, Ph.D.; Avella, Jane, B.S.; Long, Donlin, M.D., Ph.D. "EMG Biofeedback in Patients with Chronic Pain." *Diseases of the Nervous System.* 38(1977):505–9.

Hendler, Nelson, M.D.; Long, Donlin, M.D., Ph.D.; Black, Richard, M.D.; and Vernstein, Mary, Ph.D. "Diagnostic Screening Test for Chronic Pain Patients: A Selection Process for Surgery and Other Treatment Procedures." A paper presented at the second International Congress on Pain, August 1978, at Montreal.

Hendler, Nelson, M.D.; Wise, Tom, M.D.; and Lucas, Jane, R.N. "Expanded Role of the Psychiatric Nurse." A paper presented at the annual American Psychiatric Association meeting, May 1977, at Toronto. (Accepted for publication in *Psychiatric Quarterly.*)

Keiser, Lester, M.D. *The Traumatic Neuroses.* Philadelphia: J. B. Lippincott Company, 1968, chap. 13.

Kubler-Ross, Elisabeth, M.D. *On Death and Dying.* New York:

Macmillan, Inc., 1969.

Melzak, P., and Chapman, C. R. "Psychological Aspects of Pain." *Postgraduate Medicine*. 53(1973):69–75.

Snyder, Solomon H., M.D. "Opiate Receptors and Internal Opiates." *Scientific American*. 236(1977):44–56.

Sternbach, Richard. *Pain Patients' Traits and Treatments*. New York: Academic Press, 1974.

Uematsu, Sumio, M.D.; Long, Donlin, M.D., Ph.D. "Thermography in Chronic Pain." *Medical Thermography, Theory and Clinical Applications*. Edited by Sumio Uematsu, M.D. Los Angeles: Brentwood Publishing Corp., 1976, pp. 52–67.

Whistler, W. D., and Hill, B. J. "A Simplified Technique for Inspection of the Gasserian Ganglion." *Treatment of Pain*. Edited by Harold Voris, M.D., Ph.D., and Walter Whistler, M.D., Ph.D. Springfield, Illinois: Charles C Thomas Publisher, 1975, pp. 61–74.

Index